Afterglow

by the same author

Ripples in the Flow
Reflections on Vessel Dynamics in the Nàn Jing
Z'ev Rosenberg
Edited by Daniel Schrier
Foreword by Lonny S. Jarrett, M.Ac.
ISBN 978 0 85701 391 0
eISBN 978 0 85701 396 5

Returning to the Source
Han Dynasty Medical Classics in Modern Clinical Practice
Z'ev Rosenberg
Edited by Daniel Schrier
Foreword by Dr Sabine Wilms
ISBN 978 1 84819 348 2
eISBN 978 0 85701 306 4

of related interest

The Spark in the Machine
How the Science of Acupuncture Explains the Mysteries of Western Medicine
Dr Daniel Keown
ISBN 978 1 84819 196 9
eISBN 978 0 85701 154 1

Developing Internal Energy for Effective Acupuncture Practice
Zhan Zhuang, Yi Qi Gong and the Art of Painless Needle Insertion
Ioannis Solos
ISBN 978 1 84819 183 9
eISBN 978 0 85701 144 2

Gold Mirrors and Tongue Reflections
The Cornerstone Classics of Chinese Medicine Tongue Diagnosis – The
Ao Shi Shang Han Jin Jing Lu, and the Shang Han She Jian
Ioannis Solos
Forewords by Professor Liang Rong and Professor Chen Jia-xu
ISBN 978 1 84819 095 5
eISBN 978 1 84819 095 5

AFTERGLOW

Ministerial Fire and Chinese
Ecological Medicine

Z'EV ROSENBERG

Edited by DANIEL SCHRIER and
ANNE SHELTON-CRUTE

Foreword by STEPHEN COWAN

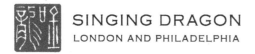

SINGING DRAGON
LONDON AND PHILADELPHIA

First published in Great Britain in 2023 by Singing Dragon,
an imprint of Jessica Kingsley Publishers
An imprint of Hodder & Stoughton Ltd
An Hachette Company

1

A CIP catalogue record for this title is available from the
British Library and the Library of Congress

ISBN 978 1 78775 412 6
eISBN 978 1 78775 413 3

Printed and bound in the United States by Integrated Books International

Jessica Kingsley Publishers' policy is to use papers that are natural, renewable and recyclable
products and made from wood grown in sustainable forests. The logging and manufacturing
processes are expected to conform to the environmental regulations of the country of origin.

Jessica Kingsley Publishers
Carmelite House
50 Victoria Embankment
London EC4Y 0DZ

www.singingdragon.com

Contents

Foreword

Stephen Cowan

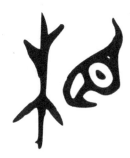

The gathering light low in trees
you can hear them flocking
in the east,

dark light in between
their cross-hatching ever more
subtle than jewels

they cluster around the shadows
as if the stars

have come home to roost.
Undrawable shapes
opposing negative space
they blend in so easily

becoming One,
fluttering in the breeze
small unspeakable ministers to the sun.
What delight da Vinci obsessed over
in backgrounds of the Florentine
or Tufu in his boat gazing out at the shore
I too here though less obsessed

delight more
in the display of day

turning inwards

this winter's morn.
SC - 12/17/19
東相火 *Dōng Xiāng Huǒ*

There is light in this book. The kind of light that comes from time well spent together. It warms the heart with its content. But context for this book matters as much as the content. Context always matters, particularly through the lens of Chinese medicine where relationships define our fundamental state of being. The unique moment in time in which Z'ev Rosenberg has written *Afterglow* is one of extreme change, both inside and out. Outside, the excesses of modern industrialization have caused global overheating, amplified weather patterns, disenfranchised and displaced people, and created political turmoil and a worldwide pandemic that has all but cut us off from each other. Inside our bodies, chronic inflammation is rising at epidemic proportions from autoimmune disease, allergies, and asthma, to disorders of anxiety, attention deficit hyperactivity disorder (ADHD), autism and Alzheimer's disease. It is as if our bodies perfectly reflect what's happening to our planet. Indeed, that is exactly what Chinese medicine has always taught. All the upheavals that stem from a rootless culture and a disembodied self are the profound impetus for Z'ev Rosenberg to write *Afterglow*.

I have had the distinct privilege of watching Z'ev methodically search through the words of the sages of Chinese medicine to help us understand how to navigate these challenging times. He is a true scholar-physician in this regard, carrying on the tradition of adapting his medicine to the particular world around him. This urge arises out of deep wisdom and compassion for being of service to people and our planet. As Z'ev points out, Chinese medicine has survived for two thousand years because it has been willing to adapt to changing times. This is what has drawn him to explore the mysteries and meanings of "Ministerial Fire" which, as you will discover, directly pertain to the circumstances we find ourselves in today.

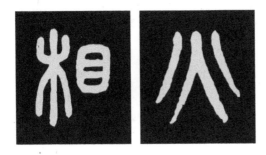

Xiàng Huǒ 相火 Ministerial Fire

At the beginning of my western medical career, I swore to first do no harm, "*primum non nocere*," only to find repeatedly that the kind of medicine I was taught in fact *does* do harm whenever it takes symptoms out of context, disregarding the subtle and complex interrelations that exist between ourselves and our environment. This is what sent me, long ago, to study Chinese medicine to find answers. The essence of our mutual interrelationships is captured in the ideogram *xiàng* 相. In it we see the image of a tree on the left and an eye on the right. I see the tree and the tree sees me! As with most Chinese ideograms, a picture is worth a thousand words and is open to many meanings depending on its context. *Xiàng* is often translated as "mutual, reciprocal, each other." But the distinct nature of Chinese characters allows them to be free to be verbs or nouns, adjectives, or adverbs. The power of *xiàng*, the tree being seen, reveals the deep ecology of mutual interdependence inherent in the holistic system of Chinese medicine. I care for the tree and the tree cares for me. Such depth of caring is what the ancient Chinese meant by being "ministerial."

In *Lǎozǐ* 老子 2 we get the essence of this *xiàng* 相 mutual dependency in a series of "each other" phrases that lie at the very core of Chinese philosophy and medicine.

有無相生

難易相成

長短相較

高下相傾

音聲相和

前後相隨

Having and not having give rise to each other

Difficult and easy complete each other

Long and short are relative to each other

High and low depend on each other

Music and voice harmonize with each other

Before and after follow each other.

The relativity inherent in Chinese perspectives is best captured by the unified *taichi* symbol of *yinyang*, the mutually generating relationship so fundamental to understanding our true dynamic nature. In this historic moment, we stand at the threshold facing the tragedy that will come from ignoring our interconnected relationships with nature. This is illustrated by the couplet *xiāng-guān* 相關 which pairs *xiāng* (each other/minister) with *guān* (a gateway/pass).

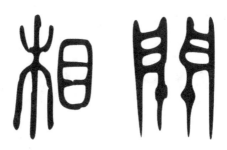

Xiāng guān is often translated as "relevancy, pertinent; to be related." When I see the tree's true relevance to my existence, suddenly my own world expands to care for the land as if it were my own body. This is the sage way of understanding our lives in context. Indeed, *xiàng huǒ* ministerial fire represents our "warm relations" for each other, whether it is the warm relations between our cells, our organs, our body and mind, or with our environment. All things in the world are our relatives. This is one of the critical messages Z'ev presents throughout *Afterglow*. When the world is on fire, I too will be on fire!

Such fire *huǒ* 火 can also be translated as "outrage," the very emotion that has charged Z'ev to write this book when he witnesses the severing of our deep connections to each other and to the planet. Z'ev is one of the pioneers of the Chinese medicine movement in the West. He doesn't just talk the talk, he walks the walk of Chinese medicine. It was by "coincidence" that Z'ev and I met at a conference a number of years ago and realized we both shared a passion for applying the classics to the times we live in. And so we became new "old friends" as he phrased it. Z'ev's previous book, *Ripples in the Flow*, offered, in concise language, new meanings to the profound nature of pulse diagnosis in Chinese medicine. This same clear communication is again here in *Afterglow*, where he explores the diverse points of view on *xiànghuǒ* held by the great masters of the past and weaves them into his own evolving perspectives on how this hidden metabolic fire pertains to the conditions we are called to treat today.

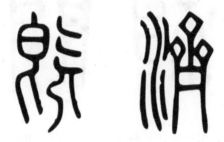

After Completion

Now that *Afterglow* is completed and in your hands, dear reader, I end with a fitting example of the multi-faceted exploration into the nature of ministerial fire in which Z'ev was kind enough to include me.

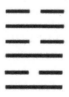

Hexagram 63

The next to last hexagram in the *Yìjīng* 易經 "*Book of Changes*" is curiously named *Jìjì* 既濟 "After Completion" or "Already Completed." It has been referenced in the classics as being related to *xiànghuǒ* ministerial fire, and Z'ev's insatiable curiosity led to several wonderful discussions with me regarding its relevance. In this hexagram, we see the fire trigram *lí* 離 sitting under the water trigram *kǎn* 坎. This is the proper way to boil water. It is the correct way to cook food, as Z'ev mentions in his chapter on cooking and ministerial fire. Thus, the next to last hexagram represents the proper place for ministerial fire to complete its duties of nourishing life. However, when the fire rises above water as we see in the final Hexagram 64, *Wèijì* 未濟, "not yet completed," the *Yìjīng* warns us that there can be no proper cooking and no nourishing of life. As Z'ev describes so well in the chapter on Autoimmunity and Thermodynamics in *Afterglow*, "when the sovereign fire in the heart is weakened, judgement and clarity of thought and awareness are clouded. When the ministerial fire flares up, it will lead to illnesses where evil heat is superimposed on yin cold accumulating in the lower burner." We see this cautionary tale today as we continue to burn up our precious resources both externally and internally. *Afterglow* should be on everyone's bookshelf to be read and reread to enable the great physician-sages of the past to guide our care for those who come to us for relief of their suffering. It is my hope that after reading this book, you will be as inspired as I have been to be the change you want to see in the world and take action.

Stephen Cowan
Autumn leaves turning red
2021

Acknowledgements

The *Rú Yī* 儒醫/Scholar Doctor as Impressionist

This book was written in the manner of an impressionist painting; like canvas in my studio, adding dabs of paint over many moons, seasons and turbulent changes in the outside world. Therefore, my apologies for any omissions of thanks.

First of all, I'm deeply grateful to my editors Daniel Schrier DOM and Anne Shelton Crute DAOM. Daniel, your dedication and continued support distilling and organizing my thoughts and ideas bring these series of teaching texts to life. Anne, your feedback as a practitioner has been invaluable. The last 18 months since the pandemic began has been a creative process collaborating through Zoom, FaceTime, and messaging in different time zones. I greatly appreciate your efforts throughout these challenging circumstances.

Next, all of my students and colleagues who gave me valuable feedback: Eti Chall, Andrea Plichta, Emily Sablosky, and Justin Penoyer, Sabine Wilms, Ken Rose, Paul Unschuld, Heiner Fruehauf, Sifu Ken Cohen, and the master of tea, Brian Kirbis, at Theasophie.

To my colleagues where I gave seminars on ministerial fire in their doctorate programs: Rob Hoffman at Yo San University, Los Angeles, Robyn Sodders at Five Branches University, San Jose, and Phil Settels at the Academy of Chinese Culture and Health Sciences, Oakland.

To Michael Max at Qiological, for his continuing inspiration and support. And a beautiful joint podcast on ministerial fire.

A special thank you to Claire Wilson at Singing Dragon Press for her patience in waiting for me to deliver the final manuscript, amidst its starts and stops, right and left turns.

A bow of gratitude to my daughter-in-law, Annie Perkins-Rosenberg, who designed the beautiful, world-class cover. It stands alone as a work of art.

A special thank you to my new/old friend, Dr. Stephen Cowan, for contributing the Foreword and collaborating on one chapter in this book. We spent the last two years since meeting at Pacific Symposium trading notes, articles, books, ideas and inspiration. Without you, dear friend, this book would not exist. Your inspiration and encouragement kept this project going during times when it appeared that the writing and preparation would never cease.

Love and gratitude to my dear wife Edith, children, and grandchildren, who make my life complete. And my rabbi, friend, and study partner, HaRav Yonatan Halevy, who continues to inspire me with new insights on almost a daily basis.

Z'ev Rosenberg,
Xiǎo Xuě 小雪, Node of Small Snow
San Diego, California, November 2021

THOUGHTS ON MINISTERIAL FIRE

Kauai Journal, February 2020

Qi is fire, fire is *qi*.
Fire follows the *qi*.
The *Sùwèn* 素問 speaks of the sun's position in the sky.
The *Yìjīng* 易經 of the orderly progression of hexagrams.
Our medical sages calculated the order of nature, in order to learn
the subtle principles that guide the movements of the heavens.
As the great feminine principle of the earth
responds, quivering in each trembling leaf,
Everything is revealed as fire and water, at its core.
Fire and water need each other, and endlessly interact in conflict,
merging, *qi* transformation, rising and falling, submerging and
ascending again, but never neutralizing each other's nature.
How can there be two fires instead of one in human life?
What were the Han dynasty sages seeing?
What stirred the interest of great European minds in
Chinese philosophy, such as Niels Bohr, Hellmut Wilhelm,
Paul Unschuld, Claude Larre and Francois Jullien? Why
did Joseph Needham, an immunologist, devote the majority
of his life to studying medieval Chinese science?

The ministerial fire ignites the yin to warm it,
enliven it, reproduce it, expand, multiply,
generate *jīng* 精/essence plus *shén* 神.
Always moving, circulating, the molten core of
human life situated between the kidneys (as described
in *Nán Jīng* 難經 66), shining in the eyes.
Warming the *shàoyáng* 少陽 qi,
warming the *juéyīn* 厥陰 blood.
Endless movement, flow and transformation.
Medical sages augmented this precious
fire with *jiǔ* 灸/moxibustion.
Aconite.
Ginger.
Cinnamon.
Stoke the *mìng mén* 命門 fire, which in
turn warms the defense qi,
And defends against cold damage where *Nán*
Jīng: "all external evils are damage by cold"
The fragility of human life is apparent
When the fire ebbs away.
But the fire also rages out of control when disturbed by
Anger.
Impatience.
Passion.
Unfulfilled desires.
Flaming up and out consuming yin, consuming essence,
"I'd give you everything I've got for a little peace of mind."
The marriage of yin and yang,
Two as one, fire and water never negate each
other, never become the same.
In Kabbalah, the mystery of creation is contained
in the unity of the opposites of fire and water.

INTRODUCTION

Occasionally, I see the world as luminous; plants and flowers shimmering in the breeze, the grandeur of sheer cliffs plunging into the sea.

Then I turn my sights to the human dilemmas of the twenty-first century, and the ecological disaster unfolding before our eyes.

Z'ev Rosenberg

The Daoists spoke of the unity of humanity and nature,[1] and how we resonate with the natural world. In the *Běncǎo Gāngmù* 本草綱目, Lǐ Shízhēn 李時珍 mentions dozens of waters, soils, and minerals as medicinal substances, each with unique and specific properties. Lǐ Shízhēn explains that our *wèi qì* 衛氣/defensive qì is a product of earth, and *gǔ qì* 穀氣/grain qì, *yíng qì* 營氣/construction qì is a product of water.

The natural endowment acquired through drinking is that of water; the natural endowment acquired through eating is that of soil. Eating and drinking are the life vessels of man; the camp and guardian [qi] depend on them. Hence it is said: Once the water is gone, the camp [qi] will be exhausted. Once the grain is gone, the

---

1 As did Oliver Sacks in the following essay: www.brainpickings.org/2019/05/27/oliver-sacks-gardens.

guardian [qi] will be lost. As it is, in the prevention of illness and the protection of life the nature and the flavor of water are to be taken into consideration.[2]

Although the United States has developed a legacy of environmentalism, through the efforts of such great men as Theodore Roosevelt and John Muir, this legacy is now endangered. There is vast damage to topsoil by agribusiness and its extractive methodology, runoff of soil, laced with fertilizers and herbicides/pesticides, into rivers, has created huge dead zones in the Gulf of Mexico, and mutagenic herbicides pollute food, soil, water, and air. Non-biodegradable plastics clog oceans and rivers, affecting fish and sea mammals. Dying coral reefs, rising average temperatures and erratic rainfall, melting glaciers and droughts are leading to mass migrations and political unrest.

In the realm of human health, the quality of food and an overload of pharmaceuticals produced by coal tar chemistry in laboratories (antibiotics, opiates, steroids, and trace substances in vaccines) has distorted the vital balance of *yīn* and *yáng*, mind and body, heaven and earth, *wèi qì*/defense and *yíng qì*/construction *qì*. Specifically, the disruption of *wèi qì* and *yíng qì* has led to an epidemic of autoimmune disorders, which we shall discuss in later chapters. At the very least, this book is the beginning of a necessary conversation that I hope will inform both Eastern and Western medical practices.

This book is the third[3] in a series of teaching texts designed to distill essential concepts and principles embedded in classical Chinese medical texts which are often left untouched in our modern

---

2   Shizhen, L. & Unschuld, P.U. (2021) *Ben Cao Gang Mu, Volume II: Waters, Fires, Soils, Metals, Jades, Stones, Minerals, Salts.* Berkeley, CA: University of California Press, p.34.

3   Rosenberg, Z. (2018) *Returning to the Source: Han Dynasty Medical Classics in Modern Clinical Practice.* London: Singing Dragon; Rosenberg, Z. (2019) *Ripples in the Flow: Reflections on Vessel Dynamics in the Nàn Jīng.* London: Singing Dragon.

schools and training courses. In this volume, we will focus on the essential substances and mechanisms of the human bio-entity, informed by the classical Chinese medical tradition, specifically, *xiàng huǒ* 相火/ministerial fire, *qì huà* 氣化/qì transformation, *jīng* 精/essence, and their role in maintaining *wèi*/defense and *yíng*/construction, the main functional qi responsible for maintaining immunity. While primarily a book about principles and foundational concepts, rather than a therapeutic and diagnostic manual, it will serve practitioners well by exposing them to classical ideas that can be applied readily to the present dilemma in the ecological crisis and to autoimmune disorders.

Xiàng huǒ/ministerial fire, dragon fire, or *mìng mén huǒ* 命門 火/life gate fire, has been an essential concept in Chinese medical texts since the Han dynasty canon. There have been different interpretations in various contexts and schools, which have often left some confusion as to the actual application of these principles. In *Afterglow*, I've investigated sources in *Sùwèn* 素問, *Língshū* 靈 樞, *Nàn Jīng* 難經, and *Shānghán Lùn* 傷寒論, as well as studying later physicians and texts such as the *sì dàjiā* 四大家/"four great physicians" of the Jin-Yuan dynasty (Lǐ Dōngyuán 李東垣, Liú Wánsù 劉完素, Zhū Dānxī 朱丹溪 and Zhāng Zǐhé 張子和), Zhāng Jièbīn 張介賓 and Zhào Xiànkě 趙獻可 from the Ming dynasty, and Zhèng Qīnān 鄭欽安 of the *huǒ shén pài* 火神派/fire spirit school, who lived near the end of the Qing dynasty. By studying this book, I hope to clear up confusion in clinical judgement as to when to supplement *yīn*, supplement *yáng*, clear heat, or clear fire.

In addition to the material on ministerial fire, I've included Lǐ Dōngyuán's perspective on qì transformation and ministerial fire. In addition, the essential subject of *jīng* 精/essence and its relationship to ministerial fire, kidney *yīn* and *yáng*, and *yuán qì* 原 氣 is discussed. Any book on a topic as fluid as ministerial fire has to be seen in the context of the various historical understandings of this functional phenomenon, as well as its modern expression and applications.

We are living through what scientists call the Anthropocene Age, where human beings have altered our planet's ecosystems beyond recognition of what they were even a hundred years ago. Chinese medicine recognizes that in order to heal society, we must heal individuals; but if society is ill, we must provide "medicine" for its disorders as well. In the *Nàn Jīng*, it says that the superior physician heals first the illnesses of society. May this book serve a small role in the healing of humanity, and the planet that we all share.

Z'ev Rosenberg, L.Ac.,
San Diego, California, Winter Solstice, 2019

CHAPTER 1

THE ELEMENTAL NATURE OF CHINESE MEDICINE

Ministerial Fire Unleashed

I. The Setting and the Stage

This chapter was started during a haze of acrid smoke, drifting up and down the West Coast from one of the worst fires ever recorded in Northern California, Oregon, and Washington. This cloud of smoke stretched from Baja, California, to British Columbia. The indigenous peoples who inhabited California, like all indigenous peoples around the world, used to initiate "controlled burns" to clear detritus, dead trees, and brush from the forests. They respected the natural cycles of our Mediterranean climate, which is wet four to five months per year, and bone dry the rest of the year. Here in Southern California, we basically have three seasons: cool/wet winters, foggy springs and early summers, and "autumn fire" season, when the land dries out, the winds blow off the desert, and temperatures climb. It is in this period when the dangerous fires occur, although due to climate change, "fire season" is lengthening, and fires are now possible at any time of year.

The essential nature of Chinese medicine reflects the experience of humans who historically have lived intimately with natural cycles, seasons, and rhythmic changes, developing a natural science and philosophy out of their observation of nature and the visible universe of stars, moon, sun and planets. Humans adapted to these cycles, learning the appropriate times to plant seeds, harvest crops, wildcraft and prepare medicines, build shelters appropriate to their environment, and harmonize with the animal, plant, insect and mineral kingdoms. It was understood that the loss of a healthy relationship with heaven and earth, with forest and plain, led to mutual destruction of the living landscape and the beings who sustained themselves on these relationships.

Chapter 3 of *Sùwèn* 素問 discusses the importance of these relationships, connecting the wellbeing of heaven, soil, humanity, and other living beings by saying:

> If this [qi of heaven] is offended repeatedly, then evil qi harms man. [Hence] this [qi of heaven] is the basis of one's lifespan. The qi of the hoary heaven, it is clear and pure, and as a result the mind is in order. If one lives in accordance with it, then the yang qi is strong. Even if there is a *zéi xié* 賊邪/robber evil, it cannot bring any harm. This [is so because one] follows the sequence of the seasons. If one misses the [sequence of the seasons], then internally the nine orifices are closed, and externally muscles and flesh are congested. The guard qi dissipates. This is called self injury; it is the deletion of qi.[1]

The ancient Chinese viewed nature and the universe as living beings, observing the expansion and contraction of natural phenomena as *qì* 氣 or "breath." These breaths informed all natural cycles, and cycles in the human organism, and built the foundations of health. This rhythmic expansion and contraction was expressed in thought, speech, and written language, and then committed to text in the philosophical and medical classics of the Qin and Han dynasties. These teachings survived thanks to

---

1   Unschuld, P.U. & Tessenow, H. (2011) *Huang Di Nei Jing Su Wen: An Annotated Translation of Huang Di's Inner Classic Basic Questions.* Berkeley, CA: University of California, pp.60–62.

a written language that transformed natural images into characters, as seen in the Chinese oracle bone script (*jiǎgǔwén* 甲骨文). Unfortunately, many indigenous cultures around the world that relied on oral transmission of knowledge were largely lost, so we are fortunate to have in our grasp a traditional medicine largely intact.

There are profound parallels and resonances between many of these ancient cultures, for example the Tibetan and Navajo cultures, when one examines their cosmologies, sand paintings, rituals, color coding, and the four directions. Navajo medicine, unfortunately, was not written down, but they had a wealth of knowledge about medicinal plants and healing ceremonies that have been recorded by anthropologists. The Chinese templates and principles recorded in the *Huáng Dì Nèijīng* 黃帝內經, *Shānghán Lùn* 傷寒論 and other medical classics spread throughout Asia, each region adapting and refining the art of healing (*yī xué* 醫學) and the medical tradition to suit their cultures, natural environment, dietary practices, and local medicinals.

It can be said that cultivating *yáng qì* through use of herbal medicine, acupuncture, and moxibustion can harmonize our patients with heavenly qì, and patients can harmonize themselves with diet, cooking techniques, use of warming "kitchen herbs" (ginger, garlic, cardamom, turmeric), and regulating sleep and activity. Since the movement of the heavens governs seasonal qì, harmonizing our lifestyles with the seasons can help preserve *yáng qì* by increased activity in summer and storage in winter time.

In Korea during the early 20th century Dr. Insan Kim Il-hoon 인산 김일훈(1909–1992), adapted five phase theory to develop a medicinal bamboo salt (*jug-yeom* 죽염). Dr. Insan would harvest his sea salt from the north shore of Korea (water phase), pack it in fresh green bamboo (wood phase), then sealed with special red clay (earth phase). These bamboo tubes are then placed in iron kettles (metal phase), which are then fired using pine firewood (fire stage).

This process is continued eight times, and on the ninth and final stage heat to a temperature of 3,092 degrees Fahrenheit, melting all the components together and producing the purest form of bamboo salt. When we examine Dr. Insan's elaborate preparation methodology we see that this was an alchemical process, based on five phase theory, that transforms minerals into medicines. Lǐ Shízhēn 李時珍 also speaks about "alchemical" preparations in his *Běncǎo Gāngmù* 本草綱目/*Compendium of Materia Medica*, in discussions on minerals such as *liú huáng* 硫磺/sulfur and *zhū shā* 朱砂/cinnabar. Repeated firing, grinding, and mixing with plant medicines can "detoxify" minerals, and allow them to be assimilated by the body more easily with fewer side effects. These methods have been adapted in medical cultures around the world such as Chinese, Ayurvedic, Tibetan, and Greco-Arabic Medicine.[2]

The same principle is expressed in *qì huà xué* 氣化學/qi transformation theory. The *wǔ xíng* 五行/five phases are all expressed in the principle of *qì* transformation as undergoing continuous circulation through a *jīng luò* 經絡/channel system "like a ring without end."[3] The key to transformation in the human being is illustrated in the relationship of water and fire. Two fires, one *jūn huǒ* 君火/sovereign fire, housed in the heart (*xīn* 心), the other, *xiāng huǒ* 相火/ministerial fire, circulating through the *shàoyīn* 少陰, *juéyīn* 厥陰 and *shàoyáng* 少陽 channels, expressing in the liver, gall bladder, *sān jiāo* 三焦 and pericardium. The sovereign fire (*jūn huǒ*) is light and illumination through the *shén* 神/spirit, and the ministerial fire (*xiàng huǒ*) is the fire of activity, movement, and transformation. These two essential fires are often distorted through imbalanced relationships with food, air, water, day and night cycles, and other human beings.

---

2   See, Liu, Y (2021) *Healing With Poisons: Potent Medicines in Medieval China.* Seattle, WA: University of Washington Press, for examples.

3   Unschuld, P.U. (2016) *Nan Jing: The Classic of Difficult Issues.* Berkeley, CA: University of California, pp.286 & 325.

All human beings attempt to self-medicate with food, drugs, sex, psychologies, spiritual practices, physical exercises, and behavior. The more extreme the imbalance, the more extreme the attempts to restore it. Without this fire to warm the body, there is no life, no consciousness, no transformation. The management of this fire is one of the major keys to health. Ministerial fire protects the body via the *wèi qì* 衛氣/defense qi, surrounding the exterior and circulating outside the channels. Ministerial fire is the warmth that transforms grain and liquid and produces postnatal qi. However, ministerial fire can flare up and burn one's *yuán qì* 元氣/source (essential) qi, as well as one's *jīng* 精/essence, when kindled by strong emotions. Its expression in *wèi qì*/defense qi can collapse, and become evil heat, which attacks the center. The ministerial fire may be consumed through "burn out," leaving the bodily vessel cold, damp, and with minimal power to transform qi and maintain life.

This is the story of life, of alchemy, transformation, longevity, health, wellness, life, and natural death. Let us once again "return to the source" and learn the keys to heal our patients, humanity, and the earth (and ourselves), by rediscovering and never losing this unifying principle.

II. Diagnosing the Ecological Crisis in America

Chinese scholars recognized that there was a yang aspect residing inside the yin earth, as well as a "ministerial fire" that transforms minerals and soil, producing gold, oil, and other precious minerals.[4] This "ministerial fire" has also transformed generations of plants and animals into fertile soil, in which crops could be grown. Alluvial soils deposited in the Central Valley of California, watered

---

4   For detailed discussion, see Shizhen, L. & Unschuld, P.U. (2021) *Ben Cao Gang Mu, Volume II: Waters, Fires, Soils, Metals, Jades, Stones, Minerals, Salts.* Berkeley, CA: University of California Press.

by mountain streams and rivers, nourished some of the richest farmland in the world.

In the new realm of the Americas, the craving for untapped resources ran wild. This lead to the consumption of natural resources, the incineration the earth's *jīng* 精/essence (oil/soil/mineral/aquifers), profiteering off the native peoples, and killing off species of animals and plants. An example of this includes Hernán Cortés and his Spanish regiment arriving in Mexico, allegedly telling the natives of Mexico that Europeans had "a disease for which gold was the only cure." Another example which followed this pattern occurred in California, as the "Gold Rush" moved west, and prosperity reigned through generations of boom and bust. The population grew, new cities spread in all directions, forests were cut, and the Central Valley of California became the "breadbasket of the world" through industrialized agriculture, with huge tracts of land mono-cropped and sprayed with pesticides. As agribusiness farming practices developed, covering huge amounts of land, streams and groundwater were depleted, and the soil was slowly destroyed by chemical fertilizers that consumed its humus content.

The same story has played out all across the globe, to the point where even formerly safe wilderness areas, such as the polar ice caps, northern Canada and Siberia, and Antarctica are now suffering from the effects of climate change at an even more dramatic rate than more populated areas. We have clearly reached the limits of sustainability. In Greek mythology, it is said that Prometheus gave the gift of fire to humanity, only to be "cursed" by Zeus to die every single day and have his liver eaten by aetos kaukasios (a Caucasian eagle). While I don't believe in the mythological gods of the Greek pantheon, there is an ironic lesson in this "gift" being used and abused as the basis of human technology. In the early 21st century, it seems as if we have reached a threshold where civilization must change course if it is to survive.

III. Ministerial Fire, Heaven and Earth: Fire and the Anthropocene Age

Normally, the weather predicts what the fire will do. In this case, the fire is predicting what the weather will do. Weather here is equivalent with *tiān* 天/heaven and the *jūn huǒ*/sovereign fire of the heart, fire below is equivalent with the ministerial fire and *sān jiāo*. Wind is associated with the gall bladder. When ministerial fire/dragon fire is dislodged from its place submerged in kidney water, the fire roars out of control and invades the heavens.

The normal cycles of heaven and earth are described in *Sùwèn* 素問, chapters 69–77, according to *wǔ yùn liù qì* 五運六氣/five movements six qi theory. The normal advance of seasons can be disturbed by *zhǔ qì* 主氣/host qi and *kè qì* 客氣/guest qi, where seasonal qi appears at the wrong time of year, overwhelms the following season, is excessive or weakened. There are multiple scenarios describing when fire, water, earth, metal, and wood qi become excessive or weakened, over-generating, and over-controlling, leading to climatic chaos. The recent addition of human influences on weather and climate, from the use of air conditioning (which adds excessive amounts of heat back into the atmosphere) to the decimation of forests, exacerbates the already natural tendencies towards chaos occurring in these cyclic patterns of year, season, node, and sixty-year cycles. Extreme burning of wood (forests) shifts wind currents and transforms air, generating evil qi. Historically, many famines, droughts, wars and social unrest, and pandemics have been generated during times of climate change. These periods were often generated by volcanic eruptions, which darkened the atmosphere with ash, changing seasonal, temperature, and rainfall patterns. The difference we see today is what many scientists call the Anthropocene Age. This period of time shows the extreme ability that humanity now has to create significant adverse effects to the Earth's climate and ecosystems, by utilizing fire to develop digital/computer technology, jet/airplane/train travel, electricity, and massive industrialized agriculture.

One of the main distinctions between humanity and other sentient beings on earth is the utilization and potential mastery of *huǒ qì* 火氣/fire qi. Fire was, and continues to be, the basis of human technology. It is our main source of energy to warm our homes, cook food, power machines, and transport ourselves across the planet. The world of pharmaceutical drugs and plastics is also the result of fire, the transmutation of fossil fuels inside the earth's crust. Human life resonates with earth qi. As a result of this resonance, what affects our health is also resonant with the health of the earth/biosphere. Human extraction of earthly fire began with rubbing sticks and stones to make sparks, which evolved to burning wood, and then digging up and burning fossil fuels, which are the *jīng*/essence of the earth. They are highly condensed plant and animal life which have transformed into a viscous mass that fills spaces in the metal and stone veins of the earth's crust, whether in liquid, solid (coal), or gaseous form. Fossil fuels are not renewable, therefore, according to Liú Lìhóng 劉力紅, the planet's interior becomes barren and cold the more we extract its yin fire from deep within its crust. The core of the earth is molten fire. The earth's interior is warmer in winter than the surface, and cooler in summer. This can be pictured as yang within yin (yang heat/fire within yin earth), yin within yang (cool yin qi on the surface of the earth).

Fire can generate its own wind, just as dry, heated wood can generate fire. If the water phase/kidney qi fail to nourish wood, wood will be dry and will ignite via wind to aggravate fire. When there is a loss of harmony with the five phases, heaven and earth qi, *yì qì* 疫氣/epidemic qi will "fill the gap" of vacuity of heaven and earth qi, and plague humanity. Heaven and earth lose communication with each other through the accumulation of toxicity in the atmosphere, bodies of water, soil, and mass death of forests, leading to a "sick planet" that in turn generates waves of illness.

The Navajo medicine men say that we have produced a "hole

in the sky" that allows pathogenic influences to descend to earth's surface. We see that fluctuations in sunspot activity, massive amounts of smoke from fires, and volcanic eruptions cause massive disruption to the atmosphere, along with large-scale use of aerosols (thankfully decreased over the last 30 years). There are untold billions of microorganisms floating through the air. The Navajo sages also tell us that destruction of natural predators allows disease-carrying rodents and deer to harbor ticks, bacteria, and viruses that spread illness.

IV. The Macrobiome and Microbiome: Medicine for Earth and Humanity

In the Han dynasty view of nature, there is a resonance among all of the natural kingdoms, including humanity, animals/birds, plants, minerals, waters, and soils. Humanity (rén 人) is seen as the conduit between heaven (tiān 天) and earth (dì 地). Our bodies and its internal environment[5] are complex systems that resonate with the earthly/heavenly realm, and are described in Chinese medicine as the jīng luò/channel system and zàng fǔ 臟腑/viscera/bowel systems. Gǎn yìng 感應/resonance is a foundational principle of Chinese medicine, expressed in clearly defined relationships between phenomena. In order to practice what Nán Jīng 難經 77 describes as "treating what is not yet ill," we must take these principles and apply them to the issues at hand.

As modern civilization has consumed our natural resources, disturbing forests, oceans, soil, water sources, and the air we breathe, the plant and animal kingdoms are disappearing. As humans consume ever more devitalized food, from soils stripped of humus and enzymatic activity, our internal "earth" has been stripped of vital microorganisms that are essential to

---

5   The milieu interieur, i.e. the internal environment or "terrain," is a concept coined by the 19th-century physiologist Claude Bernard.

transform substances from our environment into healthy qi, blood, and life.

In *An Epidemic of Absence*,[6] Moises Velasquez-Manoff, discusses the microbiome (an aspect of what Claude Bernard described as the "milieu interieur"), in terms of maintaining immunity and overall health, has central importance. Fermented foods are vital in maintaining our intestinal flora and microbiomes, and strengthening immunity and resistance to illness. Fermented foods are complex ecosystems in themselves, including such products as *pǔ'ěr* 普洱 tea, which has many different flavors, regional uniqueness, and medicinal qualities, similar to miso soup and pickled vegetables.

Infectious illnesses involving microbes such as viruses or bacteria are evolving and mutating constantly. Recent research indicates that the microbiome has a large role in building innate immunity to prevent or lessen the severity of such illnesses. In Chinese medicine, we have the principle of strengthening the *wèi qì*/defense qi and *yíng qì* 營氣/construction qi. As we have discussed elsewhere in this book, harmonizing *yíng qì* and *wèi qì* is a first-line strategy in the treatment of *wàigǎn* 外感/external contractions. The microbiome contributes to this first line of defense, and relies on microorganisms that ferment and break down food and liquids. This is what Lǐ Dōngyuán 李東垣 in his *Píwèi Lùn* 脾胃論/*Treatise on the Spleen and Stomach*[7] called the separation of *qīng* 清/clear and *zhuó* 濁/turbid qi.

We live in a biosphere permeated by microorganisms such as bacteria, viruses, yeasts, molds, and fungi, a vast majority of which are beneficial to sentient life, and maintain many of the essential functions of qi transformation in nature and in the bodies of

6   See Velasquez-Manoff, M. (2013) *An Epidemic of Absence: A New Way of Understanding Allergies and Autoimmune Diseases*. New York, NY: Scribner.

7   Dongyuan, L. & Flaws, B. (2004) *Li Dong-Yuan's Treatise on the Spleen & Stomach: A Translation of the Pi Wei Lun*. Boulder, CO: Blue Poppy Press.

plants, animals, and humans. Throughout history, Chinese medical physicians carefully observed how one's internal clock, as well as one's inner cycles and rhythms, responds to the natural world. This heavenly qi (defined as *wŭ yùn liù qì*) is expressed in yearly, monthly, lunar, solar, and diurnal cycles, along with the movement of major constellations, and is discussed in great detail in *Sùwèn*, chapters 69–77. These complex cycles can influence subtle shifts in the biosphere that can affect plants, animals, and humans and their susceptibility to disease, including *yì*/epidemics. Even today, we can observe changes in herbal prescriptions and treatment recommendations based on local climates and weather moving through warming and cooling cycles using the stem and branch transformations of *wŭ yùn liù qì*/five movements six qi theory.[8]

The Chinese physicians recognized that in *wŭ yùn liù qì*/five movements six qi theory, all sentient beings and phenomena have internal clocks which measure cycles of change: birth, growth, decay, and death. Various symptoms were recognized as being dependent on the variables of the 24-hour clock of the internal viscera, seasons, years, and other cycles, along with the flow in the vessels which could vary depending on the time of day, season, or other natural cycles. Medicinals and acupuncture points were then chosen to coordinate with the best times in regard to the rise and fall of qi. The pulse was also seen to vary at different times of day, season, or other natural cycles.[9]

In the last week or so, the southwestern United States monsoon, which is unusually strong this year, has largely replaced the usual dry winds from the southwest with a prevailing east to southeast, flow, bringing in humid, subtropical air and thunderstorms to our mountains and deserts. Since this is not the usual wind direction for our unique seasonal qi, this has brought a wave of wind/damp

8   Rosenberg, Z. (2018) *Returning to the Source: Han Dynasty Medical Classics in Modern Clinical Practice.* London: Singing Dragon, p.109.
9   Ibid., p.120.

epidemic qi, one wave being gastrointestinal, with damp/warm diarrhea, heavy mind and body, with fatigue; the other wave is primarily respiratory, with body aches, fatigue, fever, chills, sore throat and yellow to green phlegm, coughing, and sneezing. These patterns are discussed in *Língshū* 靈樞 77 in terms of seasonal qi.[10]

In the *Běncǎo Gāngmù*, Lǐ Shízhēn discusses two types of fire associated with heaven, humanity, and earth: yin fire and yang fire. On earth, yin fires are those generated by yin substances such as mineral oil (including petroleum) and which are not extinguished easily by water. In the human body, the two yin fires are ministerial fire and sovereign fire. In heaven, they are dragon fire (lightning) and thunderclap fire. Yang fires on earth include those generated by igniting wood, rubbing stones, and tapping metals. The yang fires of heaven are tàiyáng 太陽 solar fire and the "essence of the stars." They may violate earth's position through the falling of meteors, which bring heavenly fire to the surface. Many yin fires, such as those derived from gasoline, camphor, or animal fats can burn in water. Here, Lǐ Shízhēn notes:

> when one's intentions follow the Dao, and emphasize calmness, the movements of the five fires in the organism will always remained constrained, and the ministerial fire will have no other function than to benefit creation and transformation, therefore unendingly securing the engendering of life.[11]

V. The Changing of the Guard: Global Shifts, Climate Change, and Pandemics

When one studies Chinese medical history, we find an unbroken narrative of political, economic, and social changes influencing

10   Unschuld, P.U. (2016) *Huang Di Nei Jing Ling Shu: The Ancient Classic on Needle Therapy.* Berkeley, CA: University of California Press, pp.711–718.

11   Li Shizhen, L. & Paul U. Unschuld, P.U. (2021) *Ben Cao Gang Mu, Volume II: Waters, Fires, Soils, Metals, Jades, Stones, Minerals, Salts.* Berkeley, CA: University of California Press, p.119.

the practice of medicine. These changes were often in response to environmental upheavals which had occurred and in turn led to the transformation for new, innovative expressions of the core medical theories established in the Han dynasty. Within the character for medicine, *yī* 醫, we can see an aspect of the character *yì* 疫/epidemic (pestilence), thus indicating the importance of the physician in treating epidemic diseases. From the very beginning of recorded history, Chinese medicine developed strategies for treating epidemics, quite apparent in texts such as the *Shānghán Zábìng Lùn* 傷寒雜病論.[12]

In the past, climate change was driven by cataclysmic events such as large-scale volcanic eruptions spewing out clouds of ash that lowered planetary surface temperatures, reduced sunlight, and led to seasonal shifts, crop failures, and the disruption of societies. Massive population shifts often followed climate changes and the disruption to food sources, work, and political unrest that ensued. Wars, famines, and epidemics led to massive changes, which led to new eras and dynasties. The Han, Song, Jin-Yuan, Ming, and Qing dynasties each had their major shifts in agriculture practices, commerce, urbanization, and governance, and this influenced shifts in medical strategies as well.

Specific eras were more interpretive and innovative in terms of medical theory (Song, Jin-Yuan), others led back to the Han dynasty canon. But even when the *Shānghán Zábìng Lùn* and *Nèijīng* 內經 were resurrected, they were reinterpreted in commentaries that updated specific applications of the universal principles contained within. The *Nèijīng* specifically was the source of many medical currents, from the *wēn bìng* 溫病 current in the Qing dynasty to the four schools of the Jin-Yuan dynasty, including the Bǔ Tǔ Pài 補土派/Supplement Spleen/Stomach Current, Hán Liáng Pài 寒涼派/Cool and Cold Current, *gōng xié pài* 攻邪派/

---

12 At least since the Song dynasty version/compilation.

Attack Evil Current, and *zī yīn pài* 滋陰派/Nourish Yin Current. The *wēn bìng pài* 溫病派/*Warm Disease* Current also built its formulas and diagnostic strategies on the framework revealed in the *Shānghán Zábìng Lùn*, refining diagnoses and formula construction to match the new epidemics that appeared in southern regions of China during the Qing dynasty.

Currently, we are in a major transition phase, much of it caused by human activity, man-made climate change, political unrest, over population, massive pollution, and exhaustion of natural resources. We've watched as COVID-19 has transformed itself, and attacked in phases, finding ourselves as physicians of Chinese medicine obligated to apply the principles of *yīn/yáng* 陰陽, *sān yáng sān yīn* 三陽三陰/three yang three yin, *wŭxíng*/five phases and *wèi qì yíng xuè biàn zhèng* 衛氣營血辨證/four aspect pattern identification to the issues at hand, specifically when treating "post-COVID-19" patients.

Of specific importance as well is addressing constitutional types as described in *Língshū* 64 in order to understand disease susceptibility, emotional/psychological makeup, and the effects of mass migrations on human health.[13] It is this classical study that allows us to have an overview of present environmental, seasonal, and constitutional influences on disease patterns in the present day, rather than just relying on local data sources.

We must seriously consider applying the three yang three yin principles of the *Shānghán Lùn* and *Sùwèn* 素問 to emotional/psychological aspects of illness, as we are in an age of memes/thought viruses rampaging through the internet/social media and influencing large numbers of people. Conspiracy

---

13   This relates to the Bergmann's Rule, which states that animal body sizes will vary depending on the latitude and with elevation, that populations and species of larger size are found in colder environments, and species of smaller size are found in warmer regions. For more information see https://en.wikipedia.org/wiki/Bergmann%27s_rule.

theories are bred by uncertainty and people try to connect the dots of the highly complex phenomena that surround us. The "virus" of fear specifically attacks the kidney yang and heart (shàoyīn 少 陰), undermining our ministerial fire that supports our life force and immunity.

Once again, we look at the key of ministerial and sovereign fire to understand the ecological, social, and medical needs of our era. The goal of this little book is not to reinvent the wheel, but to propose new strategies for treating the disorders of our era, reframing them in the context of 2000 years of Chinese medical history.

CHAPTER 2

MINISTERIAL FIRE IN THE *SHĀNGHÁN LÙN* 傷寒論

The progressive symptom patterns described in the *Shānghán Lùn* 傷寒論/*Treatise of Cold Damage* each have corrective measures in the form of herbal prescriptions, and acupuncture or moxibustion treatments.[1] In addition, there are recommendations of lifestyle modifications in order to restore the harmonious relationship of the human entity with heavenly and earthly qi, and the harmonious movement of *wèi qì* 衛氣/defense qi (as the active expression of ministerial fire) in the organism.

Shānghán 傷寒/cold damage and *zhòng fēng* 中風/wind strike can be understood in terms of *wài gǎn* 外感/external contraction, and alternatively as a violation of the permeability of our biological, immunological, and emotional/psychological identity. There are many levels on which this can occur, but the end result is the same: debilitation of *yáng qì*, an increase of yin/cold in the body, and a decrease in the dynamic (yang) potential of one's life and health.

When we become susceptible to exterior evils *xié qì* 邪氣/evil qi, it usually means a concurrent weakening of one's *yáng qì* and

---

1   While there are suggested moxibustion and acupuncture treatments in the *Shānghán Lùn*, these are short and hardly systematic in scope. Later generations of physicians developed acupuncture/moxibustion protocols to match *Shānghán Lùn* patterns—recently Chéng Dànān 承淡安, the 20th-century Chinese physician.

vitality, and this can include our *wèi qì*/defense qi, *yíng qì* 營氣/construction qi, *xiàng huǒ* 相火/ministerial fire, *jīng qì* 精氣/channel qi, and by extension *yuán qì* 原氣/source qi. The *Shāng-hán Lùn* describes this *shāng* 傷/damage as a circular progression through six aspects of a circular movement, from the surface of the body to deep yin layers and back to the surface again. It also mirrors the rising and setting of the sun, the qi of *tàiyáng* 太陽 rising in the morning, progressing to yin stages in afternoon and evening. There is a continuous flow from yang at the exterior during daytime to the yin interior at nighttime, resembling the lung's breathing rhythms and heart's pumping rhythms.

This is expressed as *kāi* 開/opening, *shū* 樞/pivot, *hé* 合/conjoining of the *sān yīn sān yáng* 三陰 三陽/three yang three yin channels. In the yang phase, the channel progression is *tàiyáng* 太陽 (opening), *shàoyáng* 少陽 (pivot) and *yángmíng* 陽明 (conjoining/closing). In the yin phase, the channel progression is *tàiyīn* 太陰 (opening), *shàoyīn* 少陰 (pivot), and *juéyīn* 厥陰 (closing) (see figure on opposite page) *sān yáng sān yīn* 三陽三陰/three yang three yin. In the *Nán Jīng* 難經, defense qi is said to circulate 25 times during daylight hours at the exterior/yang, and 25 times in the interior/yin at nighttime. It moves with the breath, three *cùn* 寸 with each in-breath, three *cùn* with each out-breath. It penetrates all six channel stages, rising as *tàiyáng* in the morning with the sun, and being stored in the kidney just before dawn.[2] Here we see there is an essential time aspect to understanding immunology in terms of classical Chinese medicine.

---

2   See the discussion in my previous book, *Ripples in the Flow* (Singing Dragon, 2019) in the first three chapters.

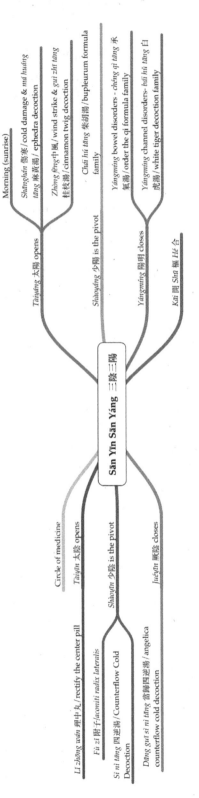

Morning (sunrise)

Shānghán 傷寒 / cold damage & *má huáng tāng* 麻黃湯 / ephedra decoction

Zhòng fēng 中風 / wind strike & *guì zhī tāng* 桂枝湯 / cinnamon twig decoction

Chái hú tāng 柴胡湯 / bupleurum formula family

Yángmíng bowel disorders - *chéng qì tāng* 承氣湯 / order the qi formula family

Yángmíng channel disorders- *bái hǔ tāng* 白虎湯 / white tiger decoction family

Tàiyáng 太陽 opens

Shàoyáng 少陽 is the pivot

Yángmíng 陽明 closes

Kāi 開 *Shū* 樞 *Hé* 合

Sān Yīn Sān Yáng 三陰三陽

Circle of medicine

Tàiyīn 太陰 opens

Shàoyīn 少陰 is the pivot

Juéyīn 厥陰 closes

Lǐ zhōng wán 理中丸 / rectify the center pill

Fù zǐ 附子 / aconiti radix lateralis

Sì nì tāng 四逆湯 / Counterflow Cold Decoction

Dāng guī sì nì tāng 當歸四逆湯 / angelica counterflow cold decoction

Sān yīn 三陰 *sān yáng* 三陽 /Three yang three yin

A large number of prescriptions in the *Shānghán Lùn* are designed to warm and regulate yang qi, in addition to protecting and supplementing the spleen qi. In *tàiyáng* disorders, medicinals such as *guì zhī* 桂枝/cinnamomi ramulus warm the defense qi, whereas in *shàoyīn*, *tàiyīn*, and *juéyīn*, *fù zǐ* 附子/aconiti radix lateralis and *gān jiāng* 乾薑/zingiberis rhizoma are employed to warm the interior. When ministerial fire accumulates in *shàoyáng* 少陽, we use *chái hú* 柴胡/bupleuri radix and *huáng qín* 黃芩/scutellariae radix to disperse and circulate; in *yángmíng*, we use *shí gāo* 石膏/gypsum fibrosum and *zhī mǔ* 知母/anemarrhenae rhizoma to disperse evil heat in the channels, and *dà huáng* 大黃/rhei radix et rhizoma and *máng xiāo* 芒硝/natrii sulfas to descend evil heat through the bowels.

I. *Tàiyáng* 太陽 and Ministerial Fire

Chinese medicine describes *wài gǎn*/external contractions as environmental excesses, although a patient with a deficient constitution may contract wind strike or cold damage from relatively minimal events, such as a blowing fan, a mild breeze, fog, or swimming in cold water. What are considered to be "physical" pathogens (viruses or bacteria) are also seen from this perspective and driven by climatic evils, winds, and weather changes. High and low pressure systems with their differentials of barometric pressure, wind direction, humidity, and temperature have a strong influence on the six paired channels in terms of sensitivity and response. Interior evils are generally classed as emotional/psychological excesses, which can increase susceptibility to *xié qì* 邪氣/evil qi as well. At the *tàiyáng* stage, immunological function is directly related to the central function of ministerial fire, and its expression in *wèi qì*/defense qi.

All externally contracted evils must navigate the *tàiyáng* channel and expel these evils through venting, sweating, or urination.

The *tàiyáng* channel is the gateway to the interior of the body, and evil qi will progress to *shàoyáng*, *yángmíng*, and eventually the three yin channels at the interior if the evil is not resolved in early stages of *tàiyáng*. Of newly contracted evils, *Fùrén dàquán liángfāng* 婦人大全良方/*Compendium of Excellent Formulas for Women* tells us that they are "tiny like autumn down feathers at the time of the violation, but more serious than the highest mountain peaks when the disease breaks out."[3] Many a minor cold has transmuted (*biàn* 變) into a more serious disorder, either by ignoring treatment at the right time, or having the wrong treatment, such as herbal formulas which do not match the condition, suppressive medications such as antibiotics or steroids, or large doses of vitamin/mineral supplements such as Vitamin C. *Tàiyáng qì* is warm, and expels wind and cold from the exterior. If not resolved, it can lodge in the *yíng*/construction/nutritive, or the *xuè* 血/blood. This warm qi that circulates through the body is identified with ministerial fire.

The *tàiyáng* great solar fire becomes indirect in winter time as the angle of sunlight lengthens as it moves south. As the calendar approaches *dōngzhì* 冬至/winter solstice (in the northern hemisphere), preserving the internal yang becomes increasingly important. It is no coincidence that in Chinese medicine the kidneys are the viscera associated with winter, the storage of *jīng* 精/essence and ministerial fire.

II. *Yángmíng* 陽明 and Ministerial Fire

Yángmíng is associated with closing and descending, and medicinal treatments will either out-thrust evil heat from the channels with cold acrid medicinals and formulas such as *shí gāo*, and *bái*

---

3   See Wilms, S. (2020) "Tinier than Autumn Down." www.happygoatproductions. com/blog/2020/1/24/itgipa6zqbivl3vqofoiqrqoez7vfw.

hǔ tang 白虎湯/white tiger decoction formula family, or downward draining herbs and formulas such as *dà huáng* and the *chéng qì tāng* 承氣湯/order the qi-coordinating formula family. In the *Shānghán Lùn*, the presence of dry stool is mentioned, and the accumulated heat dries out the *yángmíng* bowels. As *yángmíng* dryness intensifies, and the metal dry season is extended, the *tàiyīn* spleen and lung do not receive proper nourishment and lose their assimilation powers of food and air qi. Repletion patterns in the *yángmíng* (flooding pulse, abdominal fullness, thirst, heat effusion and sweating), if not resolved, will lead to the *tàiyīn* suffering from depletion. *Tàiyīn* spleen is the fulcrum of yin and yang and the central burner, and once its equilibrium is lost, (earth unable to absorb moisture), there will be extremes of dampness and dryness alternating with each other.

III. *Shàoyáng* 少陽 and Ministerial Fire

In *Sùwèn* 66 it states "*Shàoyáng* takes charge of ministerial fire" and in the *Shānghán Lùn* it states that "*shàoyáng* is the pivot." These statements have many expressions of great clinical importance, and describe the architecture of this channel as *shàoyáng* opening to the exterior/yang aspect and as a pathway to the interior/yin aspect. *Shàoyáng* opens to the east and is associated with the spring season and the emergence of yang qi from the earth to the exterior. As the pivot, this yang qi and fire pulsates, ascending and descending, constantly moving and circulating, transforming water qi via the *sānjiāo* 三焦 and circulating ministerial fire. Because of this, chronic disorders and immunological issues are often treated through the *shàoyáng* and *chái hú tāng* 柴胡湯/*bupleurum* formula family and the *hé fǎ* 和法/harmonization method. One hallmark of *chái hú* formulas is the use of oppositional ingredients, warm and cool, bitter and sweet, ascending and descending, in order to create movement out of gentle contrasts. Ministerial fire and qi then circulate throughout the channel system, the defense and construction qi are harmonized, evil heat is dissipated, and the qi transformation of water is facilitated. Because *shàoyáng* is the pivot, it often involves its adjacent channels, *tàiyáng* and/or *yángmíng*, in what the *Shānghán Lùn*, describes as a *hé bìng* 合病/combination disease.

The movement and metabolism of water controlled by the *sānjiāo*/triple burner is of great importance. Just as the earth needs to have clear, clean waterways in order for all life forms to benefit from this essential resource, our bodies flow and metabolism of water in all three burners must be harmonized, healthy, and upright. Liú Lìhóng 劉力紅 writes about "dragon veins"[4] of underground water (similar to the "dragon fire" within water of the fire trigram ☲ *lí* 離) that must be replenished, maintained, and kept clean. If we mine underground water aquifers, we further deplete the earth of its resources, leading to a loss of flow and essential yin storage factors and when we dam and pollute rivers, we destroy entire ecosystems. As humanity resides between heaven and earth, as reflections of these elemental forces our own "rivers," channels, and waterways suffer and we become ill. It is no accident that the *shàoyáng* channels are often involved in conditions that are marked by stagnant qi, chaotic movement of fire, loss of effective qi transformation, and damage to water metabolism. *Shàoyáng* illnesses are often marked by "stalemates between correct and evil qi," lingering without resolution.

---

4   Liu, L. (2019) *Classical Chinese Medicine*. (G. Weiss, H. Buchtel, & S. Wilms, Trans., H. Fruehauf, Ed.) Hong Kong: Chinese University Press, pp.359–263.

IV. *Tàiyīn* 太陰 and Ministerial Fire: The Union of Earth and Water

The *tàiyīn* chapter is the shortest chapter in the *Shānghán Lùn*, with only a few formulas mentioned, the most important being *lǐ zhōng wán* 理中丸/rectify the center pill. One explanation for this is that most *Shānghán Lùn* formulas contain medicinals such as *dà zǎo* 大棗/jujubae fructus, *shēng jiāng* 生薑/zingiberis rhizome recens, and *zhì gān cǎo* 炙甘草/glycyrrhizae radix praeparata to supplement and protect the *tàiyīn* spleen. This is similar to the *Nán Jīng* 難經, pulse chapters where the spleen qi/earth phase is seen as a specific quality of healthy pulses, but not given its own categorization as with the other four phases. Spleen/stomach qi, according to the *Nán Jīng*, is always present in the vessels, and its depletion leads to a loss of suppleness in the vessels, and an "over amplified" quality to each position. For example, wood qi is seen in a *xián mài* 弦脈/wiry pulse. If it is extreme, like the sharp edge of a knife, it is called a "visceral pulse," and is exaggerated by the lack of softening spleen qi. This reminds us of what is written above about *yángmíng* and *tàiyīn*, where the lack of moisture in the soil leads it to be dry and cracked, and unable to receive moisture or nourishment. *Tàiyīn* spleen is the fulcrum of yin and yang and the central burner, and once its equilibrium is lost (earth unable to absorb moisture), there will be extremes of dampness and dryness alternating with each other.

In recent summers in the western United States, we have seen a predominance of fire and dryness, both associated with *yángmíng*, and the metal phase of *tàiyīn* overcome by fire. This has been a progressive development over the last decade in California, as the rainy season has decreased in length (normally from mid- to late autumn to early to mid-spring), and rainfall has become more concentrated into a few intense storms, rather than lengthier, gentle rainfall over an extended period. As the mean temperatures have risen, earlier melting of mountain snows has led to heavier runoff, leading to less moisture being absorbed by the landscape. Use of aquifers and wells to provide water for intense industrial agriculture has lowered the water table below. The earth has been drying out and hardening, and cannot absorb moisture efficiently. Strangely enough the summers in the eastern part of the United States have suffered excessive dampness, humidity, rainfall, flooding, and hurricanes/tropical storms—a separation of yin and yang between east and west. *Tàiyīn*, as damp earth in a healthy state, can absorb a considerable amount of moisture. However, as in the deltas of the lower Mississippi River, too much rainfall, and paving over wetlands with concrete, can lead to flooding and damage to the earth. At the other extreme, a lack of moisture can dry out *tàiyīn* earth, leading to the inability to absorb moisture, so that it runs off into arroyos and fails to nurture plant life. It is the same in the human body: too much dampness inhibits spleen qi and its ability to separate clear (*qīng* 清) and turbid (*zhuó* 濁). *Yángmíng* extreme dryness can lead to the spleen being unable to absorb moisture, and is often connected with *xiāo kě* 消渴/dispersion thirst. In this scenario, a patient loses weight, becomes dried out with unquenchable thirst and hunger, with a thin rapid pulse, red dry cracked tongue, and sweating. This is a pattern where *yángmíng* heat damages spleen qi and essential fluids.

V. *Shàoyīn* 少陰 **and Ministerial Fire**

Shàoyīn internally resonates with *tàiyáng* at the exterior. In *Língshū* 靈樞 47, it states that "when the heart is small, then it is in peace and evil qi cannot harm it."[5] Guarding one's heart, avoiding sadness and vexation, one is protected from the attack of evil qi at the exterior. "When the heart has sunken into the depth, then the

---

5   Unschuld, P.U. (2016) *Huang Di Nei Jing Ling Shu: The Ancient Classic on Needle Therapy.* Berkeley, CA: University of California Press, p.450.

zàng 臟 lose their qi to the outside and are easily harmed by cold. They are easily made to fear by someone else's words."[6] We see this stated in *Sùwèn* 8 where it says, "If the ruler is not enlightened, then the twelve officials are in danger."[7] *Shàoyīn* is the *shū* 樞/pivot of yin, just as *shàoyáng* is the pivot of yang. Sovereign fire and ministerial fire are connected and in communication since the upper *shàoyīn* axis is the heart, and the lower *shàoyīn* axis is the kidney. As for the *wǔ yùn* 五運/five movements governance of disease, when wood, fire, earth, metal, and water all move in sequence then each is calm; when there is rebellion, then they transform into chaos, the four seasons lose their constancy, yin and yang lose balance and are conquered. This is the source of disease and was expressed in the teachings of Zhāng Yuánsù 張元素.

In *Língshū* 47, it states that when the heart is enlarged, sadness cannot harm it but it is easily harmed by (exterior) evil qi. *Shàoyīn* qi resonates with *tàiyáng* qi, which governs the exterior of the body. If *shàoyīn* qi is weak, then cold and wind evils can easily penetrate the interior. This is why strong heart qi is important to prevent even exterior contracted disorders. Professor Chén Zhìhéng 陳治 恆 believed that the most important problem in Chinese medicine was the "two roots and the three pivots,"[8] these two roots being the prenatal, relating to the kidneys, and the postnatal relating to the spleen and stomach. The three pivots are the *shàoyáng* pivot, the *shàoyīn* pivot, and the rising and falling pivot of the spleen. The "rising and falling of the spleen" is qi transformation in the middle burner. The middle burner is situated between the two fires above and below, sovereign and ministerial, and the interchange

6   Ibid., p.450.

7   Unschuld, P.U. & Tessenow, H. (2011) *Huang Di Nei Jing Su Wen: An Annotated Translation of Huang Di's Inner Classic Basic Questions.* Berkeley, CA: University of California Press, p.159.

8   Liu, L. (2019) *Classical Chinese Medicine.* (G. Weiss, H. Buchtel, & S. Wilms, Trans., H. Fruehauf, Ed.) Hong Kong: Chinese University Press, p.461.

between the upper and lower burner requires healthy spleen (and stomach) qi to raise the clear (qi) and descend the turbid (qi). Lǐ Dōngyuán, in his work, focused on the spleen and stomach as the pivot designed to activate qi transformation throughout the entire channel and viscera/bowel system.

It is interesting that the *shàoyīn* contains the sovereign ruler fire above, and that the ministerial fire is rooted between the kidneys below. It is in the domain of *shàoyīn* that the mutual interdependence and interactivity of the two fires is established. The interface of the heart's illumination and the kidney's rooting in physiological fire is what maintains *shén* 神/self-awareness, both in consciousness and physiology. The heart is able to reflect any deviation which may occur within the body with sensations of suffering. The body's self-repair mechanisms are informed by *shén*. As George Vithoulkas, homeopathic physician, said, this awareness is "like a supercomputer situated at a level which cannot be thought of in purely material terms."[9] In modern Chinese medicine, "lack of communication between heart and kidney" (*xīn shèn bù jiāo* 心腎不交) leads to forgetfulness, palpitations, night sweating, and disturbed sleep, for which *guì zhī jiā lóng gǔ mǔ lì tāng* 桂枝加龍骨牡蠣湯/cinnamon twig decoction plus dragon bone and oyster shell is prescribed.

As we discuss elsewhere in this book, the ministerial fire/ sovereign fire dynamic of heaven, humanity, and earth has been disrupted in ways that mirror the loss of equilibrium in human health, emotionally, psychologically, and physically speaking. This "gap" between heaven and earth, fire and water, inside and outside, above and below, creates a vacuum in which *xié qì* 邪氣/evil qi can flourish and disrupt life for humanity in the form of epidemics and waves of decline psychologically, emotionally,

---

9   Vithoulkas, G. (1991) *A New Model of Health and Disease.* Berkeley, CA: North Atlantic Books, p.124.

physically, and spiritually, including in our institutions of society and government.

VI. *Juéyīn* 厥陰 Disease and Ministerial Fire: Loss of Rhythmic Interchange of Yin and Yang

In this chapter on *Shānghán Lùn* 傷寒論 and ministerial fire, I have discussed how each stage of *shānghán* describes an interaction between *xié qì* 邪氣/evil qi and *zhèng qì* 正氣/correct qi. This is the dynamic interchange between cold evil and the damage to yang qi and ministerial fire, as described by Zhèng Qīnān 鄭欽安 in his work *Shānghán sùyuán jiě* 傷寒溯源解/*Exposition on the Nature of 'Shānghán."* Here, Zhèng Qīnān describes how the pathogen has penetrated to the core of yin, the *juéyīn* domain, where *sì nì* 四逆/four counter flows occur, and the limbs are cold. He states "eventually, the pathogenic qi reaches the *juéyīn* phase with its roots still intact, it reemerges into the *taiyang* and slowly over time develops into various diseases."[10] If the illness re-emerges in *tàiyáng*, if treatment is timely and correct, it can be eliminated from the exterior. If not, it will cycle again through the channels, creating a *hé bìng* 合病/combination disease of multiple (yang) channels, or a complex disease involving both yin and yang channels.

In April 2020, I was speaking with Stephen Cowan, a colleague who specializes in pediatric Chinese medicine in New York, about a phenomenon among children aged 10–15 years old called "COVID toes." Symptoms are similar to frostbite, presenting with freezing toes and fingers. I remarked that this viral attack is unusually multivalent, and this is one reason why the biomedical response has been so confused. There are different pockets of contraction,

10   McMahon, B. (2019) Zheng Qinan: Exposition on the Nature of "Shanghan," October 30. www.thewanderingcloud.com/the-archives/on-the-nature-of-shanghan.

environmental, and regional concerns, and of course different symptom patterns. A *xuè yù* 血郁/blood stasis aspect occurs in many of the symptoms we are seeing, including skin eruptions in certain cases as the body tries to vent the pathogen. This demonstrates that the pathogen in many cases directly attacks the yin channels (*zhí zhōng* 直中/direct strike) or, by passage from the yang channels, is sometimes a *hé bìng*/combination disease. In *juéyīn, xiàng huǒ*/ministerial fire warms and circulates in the blood, and the separation of yin and yang leads to a "ripple effect" of disturbance of distribution of warmth, so there is a confusing mixture of heat and cold, and the *mài* 脈/vessels are taxed. Also, cold hands and feet fall into the realm of *sì nì*/four counter flows with cold extremities, which can involve *shàoyīn* as well. So to conclude, we discussed formulas such as *dāng guī sì nì jiā wú zhū yú shēng jiāng tāng* 當歸四逆加吳茱萸生薑湯/angelica counterflow cold decoction with evodia and ginger and *guì zhī fú líng wán* 桂枝茯苓丸/cinnamon twig and poria pill among others as candidates. The clinical goal in treating *juéyīn* disease is to strengthen yang qi, descend floating yang, warm the lower burner, and circulate yin qi. We say that ministerial fire circulates in the *juéyīn* by warming and circulating the blood. The separation of yin and yang leads to a loss of binding and coordination between yin (fluid) and yang (movement and heat), and a "stuttering" quality to movement and circulation of *xuè* 血/blood. This is not unlike the "stuttering" quality to the movement and circulation of ministerial fire in *shàoyáng*, with alternating heat effusion and cold, as yin and yang are in stalemate, and one cannot overcome the other.

Stephen Cowan explains that if one let's the fire flame up (in the heart), and the water accumulate unchecked below, you have the condition associated with Hexagram 64, *wèi jì* 未濟/Before Completion, in which the ministerial fire counterflows upwards, leaving cold water below. The lower *dān tián* 丹田/cinnabar field (another name for the "abdominal cauldron" that we described in an earlier chapter) stores the ministerial fire/yang qi, and we must make every effort to center this fire in the lower burner, and not allow it to float upwards through exhaustion, emotional upset, overwork, or lack of sleep. When fire is above water, the water cannot be "cooked" or transformed. When *juéyīn* fire and water harmony are restored, then we have Hexagram 63 *Jìjì* 既濟/After Completion.

There is a similar dynamic in the relationship of Hexagrams 11 and 12. Hexagram 12 is *pǐ* 否/Obstruction (Standstill), illustrates where heaven and earth are stagnant without interaction, three yang lines (heaven) over three yin lines (earth), and associated with the autumn equinox. The nature of yang qi is to rise, and yin qi to sink. If three yang lines ascend above, and three yin lines descend below, yin and yang will not communicate. If we add the disease radical *nè* 疒, we now get *pǐ* 痞/glomus, obstruction in the middle burner, a condition of stagnant qi which inhibits movement between the upper and lower burners, the ascending of clear yang and descending of turbid yin, for which we use formulas such as *bàn xià xiè xīn tāng* 半夏瀉心湯/pinellia decoction to drain the epigastrium. Obstruction in the middle burner can also lead to failure of *shàoyīn* qi to communicate, or the pattern of *xīn shèn bù jiāo* 心腎不交/heart and kidney not communicating. Finally, if this obstruction is extreme, it can contribute to *juéyīn* disease, a complete division/separation of yin and yang. Hexagram 11, by contrast, is *tài* 泰/Great (Peace), associated with the spring equinox, with three broken lines over three solid lines, yin over yang, a time of fructification and abundance. Heaven and earth qi communicate freely with each other, and all things between heaven and earth flourish. This empty space between heaven and earth, when they are not in free and easy communication, breeds *xié qì* 邪氣/evil qi, contributing to illnesses afflicting the human, plant, and animal kingdoms. Weather becomes more extreme, great fires rage through forests, and seasons lose their regulation.

In the *Shānghán Lùn*, *juéyīn* disease typifies the rising of ministerial fire, forced upwards by yin accumulating in the lower burner, leading to heat above and cold below. This is what we call *jué* 厥/inversion. One strategy for preventing this separation of yin and yang is to practice qi gong methods to store the ministerial fire in the *dān tián* 丹田 between the kidneys, and to still the heart qi through meditation and breathing practice. Also with acupuncture and moxibustion, we can aim our treatments at maintaining open channels without stagnant qi, warming the *dān tián*, and benefitting qi transformation so that the middle burner is strong and the upper and lower burners are in full communication.

Lǐ Dōngyuán 李東垣's *pí wèi qì huà xué shuō* 脾胃氣化學說/spleen/stomach qi transformation theory is based on this strengthening of the middle qi and its ascending and descending qualities. His formulas, such as *bǔ zhōng yì qì tāng* 補中益氣湯/supplement the middle and augment the qi decoction, and *huáng qí rén shēn tāng* 黃耆人參湯/astragalus and ginseng decoction contain medicinals to raise the *qīng yáng* 清陽/clear yang,[11] and to descend fire.[12] The *huǒ shén pài* 火神派/fire spirit school utilizes formulas containing *fù zǐ*/aconiti radix lateralis and *ròu guì* 肉桂/cinnamomi cortex to penetrate and warm the kidneys and lower burner. *Fù zǐ*/aconiti radix lateralis and *ròu guì*/cinnamomi cortex also help descending errant ministerial fire down the lower burner. These observable principles of internal medicine readily apply to our understanding of the current state of the macrocosm, as with climate change.

In our present environmental crisis, we have weakened the

---

11 Medicinals to to raise the *qīng yáng* 清陽/clear yang include *chái hú* 柴胡/bupleuri radix, *huáng qí* 黃耆/astragali radix, and *shēng má* 升麻/cimicifugae rhizoma. In some variants of this formula, such as *qīng shǔ yì qì tang* 清暑益氣湯/clear summer heat and augment the qi decoction, he uses *gé gēn* 葛根/pueriae radix.

12 Medicinals to descend fire include *huáng lián* 黃連/coptidis rhizoma and *huáng bǎi* 黃柏/phellodendri cortex.

internal, ministerial fire stored in the earth through mining and consuming minerals and fossil fuels, depleted the yin aspect of earth through over-farming, over-grazing, and the use of agricultural chemicals, which are yang in nature, and "burn" and consume the yin of the soil, turning rich, loamy farmland into desert. The burning of fossil fuels makes the atmosphere turbid, blocking dispersal of contaminants, increasing surface heat, and changing wind, rain, ocean currents, and weather patterns. The altering of seasonal qi through global warming, increased droughts, areas of heavy rains, and melting ice caps has led to the burning of vital forests, already depleted by clear cutting and poor forest management.

One also needs to consider the following... in terms of *wèi* and *yíng* qi, people who have had few interruptions to their *zhēn qì* 真氣 by surgery, traumas, and multiple pharmaceuticals have a clearer vessel to self-correct and adapt to external stimuli such as pestilential qi, wind strike, cold damage, and warm disease. A person who has had multiple "suppressions of vital force" (as described in homeopathic literature) resembles a Jackson Pollock painting, lots of chaos and intertwining knots of stagnant qi and blood stasis, combined with toxicity from medications, and a poor diet.

This concludes our circular journey through the *sān yīn sān yáng* 三陰 三陽/three yang three yin theory of the *Shānghán Lùn*. As with other seminal, classical medical texts, we see that the underlying "source code" is one and the same... yin/yang and *wǔ xíng* 五行/five phases.

CHAPTER 3

SOURCE QI AND MINISTERIAL FIRE

Recharging and Rebuilding Source Qi, Defense Qi, and Construction Qi

Zhāng Jǐngyuè 張景岳 stated that the qi inside is the *yuán qì* 元氣/source qi. Whenever the physician treats a disease, they must first find out the strength or weakness of the *yuán qì*/source qi. This implies that qi transformation is an invisible process that must be understood in the context of the movements of channel qi, blood, and *jīng* 精/essence in order to comprehend disease processes, and that source qi is the wellspring of all transformations, which underlies all other substances and functions in the human organism.

My motto in treating patients, borrowed from one of Volker Scheid's teachers, is "to move a mountain with a feather."[1] When manipulating qi through acupuncture, moxibustion, or herbal medicine, one wants to be precise and gentle, being careful not to be excessive or damage the patient's qi. In order for these treatment methods to be precise, it is imperative to have a highly refined diagnosis based on *mài zhěn* 脈診/vessel discrimination.

With acupuncture, this is determined by the number of points

---

[1]   MacPherson, H. & Kaptchuck, T. (1997) *Acupuncture in Practice: Case History Insights from the West.* New York, NY: Churchill Livingstone, p.8.

that are needled, depth of insertion, strong or gentle stimulus, gauge of needles (thick or thin), and duration of treatment. A strong patient with thick musculature will need a longer time to respond, require deeper insertion, thicker gauge needles and perhaps more points needled than a thinner, yang vacuity patient with a more delicate constitution. The more precise the diagnosis, the fewer needles will be necessary. I tend to treat the *wǔ shū xué* 五俞穴/five transporting points, master/couples of the *qí jīng bā mài* 奇經八脈/eight extraordinary vessels, or choose specific channels, needling unilaterally but on opposite limbs. I then choose, if necessary, points on the abdomen or bladder/gall bladder channels on the back. Experience in practice means sensitivity to the patient's *zhēn qì* 真氣/true qi. Through palpation of the vessels, and observing how the patient's qi and emotions become centered and calm, one will know when the treatment is sufficient and not need to add excessive needles or stimulus. If we remember that the goal is not to force the qi to respond, but to gently coax it, then we will not over-treat, which will lead to less than optimal results. Because of biomedicine's emphasis on driving out disease with strong forceful medications, surgeries, and other interventions, there is a highly influential mindset that urges us to use more needles, electrostim, deep and often aggressive needling techniques. These should be reserved for acute symptoms and traumas, not chronic long-term illnesses in depleted patients.

With herbal medicine, this means using the minimal dosage, and limiting the number of ingredients to what is absolutely necessary. When prescribing herbal medicines, what I reflect on is that all stimuli, treatment, and ingestion of food and drink can be measured. I will also include mental and emotional impressions from art, media, music, news, and relationships. We should avoid trying to do too much too quickly, especially in chronically ill patients. This means not prescribing large formulas with extreme herbs that are very bitter, cold, acrid, or hot, or those that make the patient sweat, urinate, or evacuate their bowels too quickly. Many of our patients have been prescribed multiple medications, supplements, and dietary practices that overload qi transformation. I will avoid herbal treatment with a patient who has been prescribed multiple supplements, "western" herbs, medications, and treatments. In these situations, the person's qi transformation has been potentially overstimulated, and often desensitized. It is as if a computer is trying to process too much information, and slowing down in the process. Working with the patient and other practitioners or physicians, we slowly reduce treatments and medications to essential levels, simplifying the regimen, in order to allow the qi transformation to "breathe" and become more sensitive. Otherwise, it is like pouring tea into a full cup—it will only spill over the sides and on to the table.

In my practice, I favor using simple, *jīng fāng* 經方/classical formulas, one at a time. The exception is when I am treating according to season, menstrual/fertility cycles, and illnesses that require a "cyclic" approach. For example, treating menstrual problems will often require different formulas before, during, and after menses, as well as at mid-cycle. A patient with chronic insomnia may require a specific formula at bedtime, and a different formula in the morning and afternoon. For examples, please see Chapter 9, which includes a series of case histories.

The *yuán qì* 原氣/source qi is transmitted by the foot *shàoyáng* 少陽 channel, *sānjiāo* 三焦/triple burner, which also circulates ministerial fire. As it says in the *Nán Jīng* 難經, "the Triple Burner is the special envoy that transmits the original qi. It is responsible for the passage the three qi throughout the [body's] five long-term depots and six short-term repositories. "Origin" is an honorable designation for the Triple Burner.[2] Hence [the place] where [its

---

2   Unschuld, P.U. (2016) *Nan Jing: The Classic of Difficult Issues*. Berkeley, CA: University of California Press, p.473.

qi] comes to a halt is [called] "origin." In case the [body's] five long-term depots and six short-term repositories suffer from a disease, one always selects their respective [conduits'] origin [holes for piercing]." With acupuncture, one can access the source qi at the *yuán xué* 原穴/source holes on each yin and yang channel. I often debate with my colleagues that there is much more to acupuncture and moxibustion than treating musculoskeletal disorders and pain. If we use the methodology of the *Nán Jīng* and apply the *wǔ shū xué* 五輸穴/five transporting holes along with source holes, we can access the interior body, viscera, bowels, blood, fluids, and essence. When we study the *Sùwèn*, *Língshū*, and *Nán Jīng*, we see that classical acupuncture methods are clearly an integral part of internal medicine, influencing qi, blood, essence, ministerial fire, and the internal viscera.

Ideally, we are working to gently awaken *yuán qì*, sparking spontaneous healing in our patients without interfering in any way with natural intrinsic functioning. Chinese medicine has "attack strategies" for acute illnesses and situations where the damage to body and mind is too advanced to rectify without strong intervention. We can treat full-blown acute illnesses, such as respiratory infections, menstrual pain, and musculoskeletal injuries. However, perhaps our greatest calling in the 21st century is to mitigate the damage from modern lifestyle disorders, which tend to be chronic and influenced by suppressive treatment (with antibiotics and steroids), environmental toxins, climate change, and severe emotional/psychological stress. In addition, by modifying the lifestyle of our patients, we allow the source qi of the planet to be restored to its integral state as well.

As Yáng Zhēnhǎi 楊真海 states in *The Yellow Emperor's Inner Transmission of Acupuncture*, "the correct or incorrect choice of acupuncture points determines the effectiveness of Ministerial Fire in fully developing its ability to heat, move and transform."[3] This statement is very significant, and not often discussed in modern texts. I try to never forget this important principle of treatment. One expression of this is aiding the circulation of defense qi, and restoring the hierarchy in the body of defense, construction and channel qi to its normal flow and circulation.

The gall bladder is one of the channels which contains and circulates the qi of ministerial fire. As such, it is charged with balancing and stabilizing heart sovereign fire. Its central characteristic is *hé fǎ* 和法/harmonization. The ministerial fire of the gall bladder and paired channel, *sānjiāo*/triple burner, sparks all of the transformations and metabolisms of the *zàng fǔ* 臟腑/viscera and bowels. We see here that centering, sparking/enabling, and circulating ministerial fire while rooting it in the *shàoyáng* channel and lower burner (between the kidneys) is one of the foundations of health. The purpose, then, of this style of acupuncture treatment is to restore the source qi, center the ministerial fire, and restore integrity to the body and mind. "Moving a mountain with a feather" means finding the most subtle, precise, and gentle treatment that will gently awaken the body/mind memory and restore health without undue force.

The needs of my patients shifted away somewhat from specific complaints to an overall need to recharge, rebuild, and connect with their own source qi, correct qi, and defense qi. In my clinical practice, I subtly shifted focus with the onset of the COVID-19 pandemic. After some preparation time creating a safe office environment, I decided to treat only one patient per hour. Based on my studies of source qi and ministerial fire while researching this book, I decided to work in a more subtle yet focused manner, aiming to enhance the source qi and facilitate harmony of *wèi qì*

---

3   Zhenhai, Y. *et al.* (2019) *The Yellow Emperor's Inner Transmission of Acupuncture.* Hong Kong: Chinese University Press, p.35.

衛氣/defense and *yíng qì* 營氣/construction qi. I took into account five phase dynamics, yin and yang channels, chronobiology, vessel palpation, and tongue analysis.

I rely on distal *xué* 穴/holes on specific acupuncture channels according to the three yang three yin channel differentiation described in *Sùwèn* 31 (*Rè Lùn* 熱論/*Treatise on Heat*), and the *Shānghán Lùn* 傷寒論. I also apply treatment to the extraordinary vessel master/couple points, *wǔ shū xué*/five transporting points chosen according to five phase theory, along with "local points" on the abdomen (*mù xué* 募穴 alarm points) and the back *shù* points (*bèi shù xué* 背俞穴).

In terms of herbal formulas, depending on which channels are affected, and the relationship of *yíng qì* and *wèi qì* 衛氣, I rely on the formula families first recorded in the *Shānghán Lùn*. Each of the three yin and three yang channel patterns, individually or in combination, has a family of formulas that apply to the symptom pattern as it evolves. In complex cases, multiple channels may be involved, and what the *Shānghán Lùn* describes as *hé bìng* 合病/combination diseases, where more complex or modified formulas may be necessary. For example, a simple *shàoyáng* disorder would use the "flagship formula" *xiǎo chái hú tang* 小柴胡湯/minor bupleurum decoction. However, if there are also symptoms of *tàiyáng* 太陽 disease, we would combine *guì zhī tāng* 桂枝湯/cinnamon twig decoction with *xiǎo chái hú tāng*/minor bupleurum decoction, creating a new formula, *chái hú guì zhī tāng* 小柴桂枝湯/bupleurum and cinnamon decoction. If the pattern involves sweating, glandular swelling, heat effusion, and lung involvement, we may choose a further modification, *chái hú guì zhī gān jiāng tāng* 柴胡桂枝干姜汤/bupleurum, cinnamon twig and dried ginger decoction.

In the *Zhēnjiǔ jiǎyǐ jīng* 針灸甲乙經/*Systematic Classic of Acupuncture and Moxibustion*, Huáng Fǔmì 皇甫謐 speaks about the needling method of *tōng jīng* 通精/communicating essence.

This technique employs a slow, subtle insertion of needles, and careful removal (after a minimum of 28.5 minutes, according to the *Nán Jīng*). Supplementation and drainage of specific holes and channels is not handled mechanically by lifting, thrusting, or pointing the needle with or against the channel. Instead, one finds the "sweet spot" at the interface between the *wèi*/defense and the *yíng*/construction, and it is here where yin and yang can be harmonized, qi flow enhanced, and equilibrium restored. We can also conclude that channel qi flows at this interface between *yíng qì* and *wèi qì*.

We need to aid our patients' efforts to rebuild and connect with their own source qi. The atmosphere of uncertainty, relative isolation, and vulnerability to a hidden pathogen has had a definite influence on patient needs, and I adjusted my style of practice accordingly. Now that the acute threat of the pandemic has lifted to some degree at the time of writing this book, I find my style of practice is still the same. Ironically, new viral epidemics are spreading across the country at the peak of summer (between *xiaoshǔ* 小暑/small heat and *dàshǔ* 大暑/great heat, mid-July), and new variants of the COVID-19 virus continue to affect pockets of the country.

We can summarize that careful vessel diagnosis, palpation, and choice of herbal formulas and acupuncture based on these principles provide the Chinese medicine practitioner with a sophisticated toolset for our modern "palate" seen in clinic of complex, chronic, and autoimmune disorders. We carefully rebuild our patients' source qi with full focus and intent, utilizing time to create a better future.

CHAPTER 4

DEFENSE QI, CONSTRUCTION QI, AND MINISTERIAL FIRE

A Survey of Classical Sources and Commentaries

Biomedicine uses what I consider to be an "engineering" model to explain the immune system, based on the interaction of specific molecules (T-cells, antibodies) and pathogens (viruses, DNA/RNA, bacteria, spirochetes). These interactions and responses are catalogued according to the view that the immune system has a "library" of catalogued pathogens, responsive structures, and mechanisms developed over a person's infectious disease history. This is a useful approach towards a practical understanding of immunology, especially in epidemics where specific pathogens are targeted, but this engineering model applied to the complexity of organic human life has limitations. Because of its overwhelming complexity, it is difficult to find a systems approach and unified theory for immunology within the biomedical paradigm. Much of the detail and complexity is still unknown or poorly understood, as we've seen with the unpredictability associated with the COVID-19 pandemic and the immune response to this specific coronavirus. One alternative model that was offered was the Immune Network Theory of Francisco Varela. The famous Chilean scientist, philosopher, and neurobiologist viewed the immune system as a cognitive, intelligent network, and as "a self-referential system made up of mutually interacting molecules" and proposed that "the immune system is a genuine cognitive system, which despite the probabilistic character of its intercellular connections can support processes like memory, learning, self and recognition."[1]

By contrast, Chinese medicine uses a "systems approach" and complexity, seeing the macroscopic view as essentially including seasonal qi, climate, human activity, emotions, age, constitution, immune history (*wài gǎn* 外感/external contractions and *nèi shāng* 內傷/internal damage), and other factors in designing responses.[2] Zhāng Dōng 张东, in his book *Yuánqì shén jī* 元氣神機 explains it as follows: "the root of treating illness ought be allowing the 元氣 original qi of the body to heal without action."[3] In our present era of climate change, pandemics, and social upheaval, it is essential to cultivate and harmonize original qi through self-acupuncture/moxibustion, herbal medicine, healing diet, qi gong/yoga, meditation, prayer, and long walks in nature. While during epidemics *gōng xié* 工邪/ attacking evil (qi) may be necessary as part of a therapeutic response, along with social measures such as distancing and isolation, we can enhance and provide a foundation for those efforts by securing our own health and source qi through daily practices.

Língshū 靈樞 66 states:

When a depletion evil strikes a person, in the beginning it is in the skin. When the skin is relaxed, then the skin structures are open.

1 Bartłomiej, S. (2019) "Francisco Varela's Vision of the Immune System." *Ruch Filozoficzny*, 75(2), 209.

2 The modern discipline of systems biology, along with related disciplines such as complexity theory, provide more suitable modern interfaces with the systems approach of Chinese medicine.

3 Farquhar, J. (2020) *A Way of Life: Things, Thought, and Action in Chinese Medicine.* New Haven, CT: Yale University Press, p.133.

When they are open, the evil qi enter via the body hair. Once they have entered, they proceed into the depth.[4]

Cold, and the progression of *shānghán* 傷寒, is seen by such physicians as Zhèng Qīnán as the weakening and debilitation of the body's yang qi, which expresses itself both as defense qi and ministerial fire.[5] Wind strike and cold damage enter the body through the *tàiyáng* 太陽 channel (wind affecting the defense qi, and cold the construction qi). When yang qi is debilitated, qi transformation is impaired, allowing exterior evils to lodge in the channel and gradually penetrate the channel system to the deep yin layers. This chapter continues by describing how the body "stores" evil qi as *shānghán* 傷寒, progresses to the interior, and settles in the *mó yuán* 膜原/membrane plane (source). This cold evil can attack from the *còu lǐ* 腠理/interstices (the spaces in the skin), or from below via the foot yin channels. *Sùwèn* 31 and the *Shānghán Lùn* 傷寒論 systematized this progression in terms of three yang and three yin channel/warps, whereas the *Língshū* saw it more in terms of penetration of network vessels, main "conduits," and the extraordinary vessels.

In the summer time, as heat and humidity increase, human beings seek coolness through fans, air conditioning, and cold foods and beverages. However, in summer the pores are open, and people sweat in order to vent excessive heat. The open pores can allow cold and damp to penetrate the *tàiyáng* 太陽 channel through exposure to air conditioning, fans, or sudden cooling temperatures by swimming in cold water, sleeping directly under fans or vents, or getting drenched in thunderstorms. This can lead to "summer

---

4   Unschuld, P.U. (2011) *Huang Di Nei Jing Ling Shu The Ancient Classic on Needle Therapy*. Berkeley, CA: University of California Press, p.605.

5   See McMahon, B. (2019) *Zheng Qinan: Exposition on the Nature of "Shanghan,"* October 30. www.thewanderingcloud.com/the-archives/on-the-nature-of-shanghan.

colds," which are difficult to treat as they are not "*zhèng* 正/correct" seasonal evils.[6]

In *Sùwèn* 69, Wáng Bīng 王冰 states:

> The three yin and the three yang control heaven and earth. It is through them that the arrangement of the generation and transformation of yin and yang is manifested. That is called: "Positioned in heaven and positioned on the earth." The five periods reside in the center; they govern the changes and transformations of the human qi. Hence [the text] states, "Penetrated by the human qi."[7]

Here, we see the cosmological foundations of both san yang/san yin theory and *wǔ xíng* 五行/five phase theory. These were adapted in Chinese medicine to create effective immunological maps to guide diagnosis and treatment of both external contraction and internal damage disorders.[8] Yáo Shàoyú 姚紹虞 also states that:

> The qi of heaven, earth, and man have their fixed position. That is their *běn* 本, "base." The "line patterns of heaven" include the stars and the other heavenly bodies, wind, rain, cold, and summer-heat. Their qi is based in heaven; it is positioned above. The "structures of the earth" include mountains, rivers, birds, fishes, animals, and plants. Their qi is based on the earth; it is positioned below. The "affairs of man" include qi and blood, depletion and repletion,

---

6   Each season has its "correct" pathogen/evil, corresponding to the predominant climate in that season. So in summer time, heat is a "correct" evil. Cold is a "correct" evil for *dōng* 冬/winter. So exposure to cold in the summer time leads to a more complex illness than in the winter time.

7   Unschuld, P.U. & Tessenow, H. (2011) *Huang Di Nei Jing Su Wen: An Annotated Translation of Huang Di's Inner Classic Basic Questions*. Berkeley, CA: University of California Press, p.243.

8   Five phase theory and internal disorders will be discussed in depth in my forthcoming (early 2024) *Nán Jīng* 難經 commentary text on the treatment of disease, entitled *A Ring Without End*.

outside and inside, countermovement and obedience. Their qi is based in man; it is positioned in the center."[9]

Here we see the convergence of heaven and earth qi, heaven qi descending from above, earth qi rising from below, with humanity at the center, serving as a conduit between heaven and earth, but also under influence from above and below in terms of health. It is impossible to separate the health of human beings from the conditions in the heavens and on the earth. Medicine is a meditation on the cosmos and ecological integrity of the earth and cannot be separated from these concerns. This is the great message of the *Huáng Dì Nèijīng Sùwèn* 黃帝內經素問.

The authors of the Chinese medical classics understood that the illnesses of humanity have a direct correspondence with the "illnesses of earth," which in turn are caused by aberrations of the *wǔ yùn liù qì* 五運六氣/five movements and six qi, season, year, constellations. Yin and yang lose their mutual balance and flow, creating disturbances that can affect weather, climate, seasonal qi, agriculture, environmental factors, and human health.

---

9   Unschuld, P.U. & Tessenow, H. (2011) *Huang Di Nei Jing Su Wen: An Annotated Translation of Huang Di's Inner Classic Basic Questions.* Berkeley, CA: University of California Press, pp.243–244.

CHAPTER 5

THOUGHTS ON SUPPLEMENTING YANG QI

I. Preserving Ministerial Fire

At summer solstice, the yang qi begins to decline towards yin. On the circle of ascending yang and descending yin, this marks the return towards winter which we can see in Hexagram 44, *gòu* 姤/Temptation.[1] In terms of human life, this also marks the time when yang qi and ministerial fire begin to decline. As such, it is an important time to replenish and preserve yang qi in order to optimize qi transformation and maintain defense qi, digestion, and the essential functions of the body. Ministerial fire metabolizes the yin essences of the five *zàng* 臟/viscera, so this is one of the situations where we supplement yin, blood, and/or *jīng* 精 by supplementing yang qi.

Zhāng Jingyuè 張景岳 states that there is a natural order of generation and decay of yang qi which supports the life and death of all living things. In terms of *yǎngshēng* 養生/nourish life and longevity, human beings who wish to live their optimum lifespan without decrepitude must resist this tendency in the "autumn of their life" to allow yang qi to decay. This implies that simply "following the natural order" is not the Dao of health. As Zhāng

---

1 *Gòu* can be translated as "meeting" or "encountering." It is the image of *qián* 乾/heaven over *xùn* 巽/wind, and has the image of wind blowing down a mountain.

Jingyuè states, "can one allow the river of time to pass by without aspiring to be a firm rock (in midstream)?"[2]

A key to safeguarding health in wintertime (dōng 冬) is to create a core of yang, warmth, a "fireplace" that stores ministerial fire. In traditional Japanese and Korean homes, there are hearths set into the floor, with a cooking fire and tea or soup. Traditional houses did not have central heating, so historically the Japanese, when they ate their meals, would sit on the floor with their legs under low tables (kotatsu 炬燵) heated with wood charcoal. In addition, tiny charcoal burners were worn on the lower abdomen (dān tián 丹田) to maintain the warmth of the abdominal cauldron. Once cold evils penetrate the yin channels, warm to hot medicinals and formulas and moxibustion treatment are necessary. Once wind or cold evils reach the yin channel domains, the ministerial fire has been weakened, as the yang channels work to keep exterior evils from entering the interior. Ministerial fire can be eroded by too much consumption of cold food or beverages, the aging process, insufficient clothing or a heating source, using cold formulas and herbs, exposure to air conditioning, and repeated contractions of shānghán 傷寒 or zhòng fēng 中風.

We see that regulation and circulation of ministerial fire and its expression as defense qi is a major part of treatment strategies in the Shānghán Lùn 傷寒論, and that this concept of vital heat is central to understanding the diagnosis and treatment of disease in Chinese medicine. As our yang qi begins to decline with age, we should treat ourselves with moxibustion and yang medicinals such as fù zǐ 附子/aconiti radix lateralis, gān jiāng 乾薑/zingiberis rhizoma, ròu guì 肉桂/cinnamomi cortex, as well as essence-supplementing medicinals such as the medicinal mushrooms (líng zhī 靈芝/ganoderma, dōng chóng xià cǎo 冬蟲夏草/cordyceps, xiāng

---

2   Jingyuè, Z. & Tsaur, A. (2020) *Complete Compendium of Zhang Jingyue Vol. 1–3.* Middletown, DE: Purple Cloud Press, p.256.

gū 香菇/shitake, *bái huà rōng* 白桦茸/Chaga), *rén shēn* 人參/ginseng radix and *yù zhù* 玉朮/polygonati odorati rhizoma. Formulas such as *dāng guī sì nì jiā wú zhū yú shēng jiāng tāng* 當歸四逆加吳茱萸生薑湯/tangkuei decoction for frigid extremities plus evodia and fresh ginger, *fù zǐ lǐ zhōng wán* 附子理中丸/aconite accessory root pill to regulate the middle, *zhēn wǔ tāng* 真武湯/true warrior decoction and *shèn qì wán* 腎氣丸/kidney qi pill are significant in this stage of life.

Qi gong, yoga, walking and light physical activity are important to allow for qi transformation. Cooking foods which are easily digested such as whole grains (millet, kasha, black rice, quinoa), beans (adzuki, lentil, black bean), seasonal and fresh vegetables and fruits along with small amounts of animal protein if required (fish or organic chicken), while being careful with sweets, dairy products, raw vegetables and fruits, and especially iced or cold foods and drinks, is of great importance. Aging is a lifestyle, and if one does not cultivate one's own health, one will be forced to engage in the "biomedical lifestyle" of multiple doctors' appointments, multiple medications and procedures, and limitations on one's daily activities.

II. Cooking and Ministerial Fire

Every few years, a new dietary fad takes hold—The Raw Foods Diets, Atkins, Cambridge, South Beach, Keto, and periodic fasting—all of them having some merit but none of them based on the traditional wisdom that informs cultures that live with heaven and earth on a daily basis. *Sùwèn* 素問 specifically contains theories of balance of flavors in food and medicine. Each food has a refined essence expressed as flavor, which targets specific phases and associated viscera and bowels. This in turn can be modified by cooking, pickling, and appropriate seasoning, in addition to creating harmonious combinations of flavors, textures, and qualities with other foods. Adding external fire from different kindling and modifying further with cooking vessels, intensity of heat, use of warming spices, and length of cooking times, are all methods of enhancing the ministerial fire of human beings and yang qi. The yang qi is the root of separation of clear and turbid qi, generating qi and blood, circulating floods, and maintaining defense qi and bodily warmth. In wintertime, use of more dense, warming foods (roots, barks, and seeds) and longer cooking techniques in stews and baked dishes are good to increase storage of yang qi and ministerial fire in the *dān tián* 丹田. In the summer, the use of more leaves, flowers, and fruits with lighter cooking methods is preferred. Lǐ Shízhēn also emphasizes the importance of food preparation by stating:

> The extent to which the preparation of food is based on fire is related to the [people's] illnesses and diseases and longevity, to their dying young and surviving [until a late death]. As long as, in the course of the four seasons, tinder wood is drilled to obtain a fresh fire which then is used to prepare beverages and food, and as long as excesses and shortages are avoided by acting in accordance with the [changing nature of] qi in the course of the four seasons, the people are protected against those illnesses that are associated with [the qi of] the seasons.[3]

III. Traditional Cooking Methods and Ministerial Fire

As food is the major source of qi, how we prepare it is of extreme importance to our health. Human technological acumen has allowed us to harness fire to prepare our food in different ways,

---

3   Shizhen, L. & Unschuld, P.U. (2021) *Ben Cao Gang Mu, Volume II: Waters, Fires, Soils, Metals, Jades, Stones, Minerals, Salts.* Berkeley, CA: University of California Press, pp.119–120.

some preferable to others. Just as with the preparation of herbal medicinals by *duì yāo* 對么 and *páo zhì* 炮製, foods are modified through various preparation methods to enhance their health-giving qualities and combinations. These include:

- pit roasting: burying foods and herbs in the ground, basically covering them with earth and using hot coals from consumed firewood

- wood fire: including wood stove cooking

- using ox manure as fuel (prevalent in the Himalayas, where wood is often scarce)

- peat fire (common in Ireland)

- rice straw—rather than burning off fields, rice straw can be used as cooking fuel

- baking in clay ovens.

Each of these methods, using natural fuels, is environmentally sound and nurtures fire with slow, deliberate cooking. The *Běncǎo Gāngmù* 本草綱目 mentions four types of wood associated with each season that are appropriate for cooking: elms and willow in spring time, apricot and date tree wood in summer, xylosma in autumn, sephora and sandalwood in winter, and maclura and mulberry heart wood corresponding with the spleen/earth transitions of earth.

We can also see, in the evolution of technological advances, that new methods of cooking have also been developed: gas stoves, electric stoves, and microwaves. Both electric stoves and microwave ovens rely on electrical impulses to cook food, a very indirect method of generating heat when compared to using true fire. In addition, the qualities of foods can be modified through fermentation/picking, and using miso as external replication of the human digestive system. Specifically, in the *Nán Jīng* 難經, the middle burner is compared to a compost pit, where fermentation occurs to allow assimilation and separation of clear and turbid qi.

Cooking vessels also modify and influence the quality of food. Food absorbs the qi of both the cooking fuel and the vessel in which it is cooked. The quality of the metal or earthenware/ceramic base that is used influences both the qi and flavor of the food. From the most precious metal (gold) through to modern synthetic materials such as teflon used in "non-stick" pans, we cannot afford to ignore how synthetic materials may subtly poison the food and actually siphon nutrients out as it cooks. Examples of materials used for cooking vessels include gold, copper, cast iron, earthenware, stainless steel, and teflon. With the exception of stainless steel, all of the above materials can permeate the food to various degrees, depending on length of cooking time, ingredients such as spices, and porosity. This, of course, is especially dangerous with teflon, a synthetic product (plastic), which can allow toxic substances to mingle with the foods. The cooking of food is an interaction between raw food materials, cookware, source of heat/fire, along with intensity of heat and time on the fire, all influencing the outcome of the food. The skillful addition of fire to food has an alchemical effect that can not only provide nourishment, but feed the ministerial fire and spleen/stomach qi.

CHAPTER 6

AUTOIMMUNITY AND THERMODYNAMICS

I. Management of Ministerial Fire to Maintain Equilibrium

In the modern clinical practice of Chinese medicine, we often encounter many patients with chronic, complex disorders, such as multiple sclerosis, lupus, allergies, chronic fatigue, gynecological disorders, asthma, arthritis, and cancer. Many practitioners find their diagnoses lacking consistency, tending to excessive simplification of the diagnosis, and an inability to organize clinical information coherently. This is potentially the result of over-reliance on *zàng fǔ biàn zhèng* 臟腑辨證/bowel and viscera pattern differentiation, a "snapshot" diagnosis which tends to fix the illness in a static location. Most chronic illnesses involve multiple visceral systems and patterns, meaning a more elegant approach to diagnosis is necessary. *Zàng fǔ* pattern differentiation and *bā gāng* 八綱/eight principle pattern differentiation are excellent in locating the present position of an illness, but less useful in tracing the origins and continuing development of these disorders.[1]

---

[1] *Bā gāng biàn zhèng* 八綱辨證/eight principle pattern differentiation is based on the work of Zhāng Jingyuè's *Jingyuè Quánshū* 景岳全書, but is greatly simplified from his description in that text. For reference, see Jingyuè, Z. & Tsaur, A. (2020) *Complete Compendium of Zhang Jingyue Vol. 1–3: Eight Principles, Ten Questions, and Mingmen Theory*. Middletown, DE: Purple Cloud Press.

Thermodynamics is a branch of physical science that deals with the relationship between heat and other forms of energy (such as mechanical, electrical, or chemical energy), and, by extension, of the relationship to all forms of energy. I've reframed this technical term from modern physics in the context of Chinese medicine. Namely, it describes how vital heat as an expression of yang qi is transformed and transported throughout the human organism by the *sānjiāo* 三焦/triple burner. Understanding "thermodynamics" in Chinese medicine means understanding the principles of *xiāng huǒ* 相火, *jūn huǒ* 君火, and *mìng mén* 命門. The currents of supplementing yang, fire spirit, and cold damage all emphasize the importance of yang qi. The *wēn bǔ xué pài* 溫補學派/warm supplementation current utilizes warm medicinals such as *fù zǐ* 附子/aconiti radix lateralis, *gān jiāng* 乾薑/zingiberis rhizoma and *ròu guì* 肉桂/cinnamomi cortex to warm the yang and supply vital heat that is circulated through the channels, blood, and fluids of the body, largely via *sānjiāo*/triple burner dynamics.

In Chinese medicine, the inflammation associated with auto-immune disorders can be understood and reframed as the floating and drifting of errant ministerial fire through the body, combined with loss of regulation of the *wèi qì* 衛氣/defense and *yíng qì* 營氣/construction qi. The ministerial fire is displaced by accumulation of cold and damp in the lower burner. If exterior cold penetrates the *tàiyáng* 太陽 and sinks, it will start to impact the channels, fluids, blood, and viscera. Zhāng Jǐngyuè 張景岳 states:

> When yin prevails in the *mingmen*, the original yang will flee due to fear. As the dragon fire no longer has a place of refuge, it will roam and wander without returning to its source; as a result there will be diseases such as heat vexation and repelled yang. When one's intentions follow the orders [of the Dao] and in addition emphasize calmness, the movements of the five fires [in the organism] will always remain constrained, and the minister

fire will have no other function than to benefit creation and trans-formation, thereby unendingly securing the engendering of life. How could it be a robber [of the original qi]?[2]

Zhū Dānxī 朱丹溪 similarly states that "huǒ 火/fire stirs by wàng 望/hope, expectations."[3] This is based on society's expectations, having to create a false persona, not following one's heart in choice of home, marriage, relationships, work, or conflicting desires.[4]

Here, we can see that the ministerial fire's association with gall bladder qi has a dynamic relationship with the sovereign fire of the heart. When the heart qi becomes scattered by emotional exhaustion and distraction, one's attention becomes devoid and results in what biomedicine defines as "attention deficit hyper-activity disorder (ADHD)." In Chinese medicine, this is seen as scattering of the shén 神 and sovereign fire, and the gall bladder's ministerial fire will be unleashed. The emperor is no longer rul-ing from his throne, centered in the chamber of the heart, so the minister runs wild, igniting "small fires," and leaving other parts of the channel system cold and depleted. This leads to chaos of yin and yang, yíng and wèi. A reverse pattern can also occur. When the heart becomes overcome by emotional overload and an excess of information, the gall bladder as rectifier grounds and centers the heart, restoring balance. Appendix II discusses the formula dìng zhì wán 定志丸/settle the will pill, and its relation to treating this issue.

When I was a child, my favorite movie was Walt Disney's Fan-tasia, specifically the section on "The Sorcerer's Apprentice." The

---

2   Jingyuè, Z. & Tsaur, A. (2020) Complete Compendium of Zhang Jingyue Vol. 1–3. Middletown, DE: Purple Cloud Press, p.309.

3   Can be additionally seen as entitlement, falsehood, egotism, and presumptuousness.

4   Scheid, V. (2016) Desires: Capitalism, The Pope and Chinese Medicine. March 26, http://somatosphere.net/2016/desires-capitalism-the-pope-and-chinese-medi-cine.html.

magician's assistant, played by Mickey Mouse, has command of his "servants," who are brooms that sweep the floor, and buckets that carry and pour water. When the master magician is away, the apprentice tries to command the brooms, mops, and buckets, and soon they get out of control. They not only multiply in their numbers, they fulfill their role chaotically, leading to flooding of the sorcerer's headquarters. At the end of this section of the movie, the sorcerer reappears to establish the lost order that occurred when he left the scene. In a similar manner, ministerial fire and defense qi attempt to expel wind and/or cold evils from the body, but if these defense mechanisms are not successful, they will end up accumulating, inflaming, and creating an oppositional dynamic of yin and yang, heat and cold, with an increasing complexity of symptoms.

When the sovereign fire in the heart is weakened, judgment and clarity of thought and awareness are clouded. When the ministerial fire flares up, it will lead to illnesses where evil heat is superimposed on yin cold accumulating in the lower burner. This is why consumption of yin, cold foods and drinks, ice, and cold medicines such as antibiotics, steroids, and many vaccines damage yang qi, allowing yin cold water to accumulate in the lower burner, in turn leading to ministerial fire moving chaotically through the channels. This can be seen in many of the symptom patterns associated with such illnesses as lupus erythematosus, where sudden skin eruptions, drying of the eyes and mucosa, mental confusion, swelling, and pain can occur.

The emotion associated with yin cold in the lower burner is fear—fear of aging, fear of illness, fear of death, "the great yin." During menopause (andropause in men), the lower burner becomes more cold and damp, leading to a disharmony between heart and kidney in *shàoyīn* 少陰, with cold/damp pushing up the ministerial fire. In modern Chinese medicine practice, this is often misinterpreted as kidney *yīn* vacuity fire, and the *yīn* is supplemented with *liù wèi dì huáng wán* 六味地黃丸/six flavor rehmannia pill. However, if one checks the pulse (*yīn xū* pulses are thin deep and rapid for the most part), tongue (*yīn xū* tongues are red, peeled, and/or shriveled) and abdomen (in most cases, the abdomen will be soft and cold when *yáng xū*, tense and hot when *yīn xū*), these signs can confirm the diagnosis.

II. Essential Questions in Understanding Ministerial Fire and Autoimmunity

1. What is *yíng qì* 營氣 and *wèi qì* 衛氣?

The relationship of *yíng qì*/construction to *wèi qì*/defense qi is one of the most important principles in Chinese immunological approaches. This particular expression and dynamic of yin and yang defines the relationship of exterior/interior, warmth qi and fluids, skin and tissues, ministerial fire and *yuán qì* 原氣/source qi.

2. What is *shén* 神/spirit?

In the context of this book, *shén* is awareness of one's own body and emotional state, and the conditions of symptom clusters, sensation or lack of sensation, warmth and cold, presence or lack of awareness.

3. What is *jīng* 精?

Jīng is activated yin, with a spark of yang qi. It is the storage capacity of the internal yin viscera, specifically the kidneys. This stored essence is activated by ministerial fire to support the organism, and is an essential component of the physical constitution.

4. What is the relationship of *yíng qì* and *wèi qì* in autoimmune disease?

Nán Jīng 難經 30 sums this up: "The construction and guard qi follow each other. The yin and yang conduits are tied to each other like a ring without end."

5. What is *zhèng qì* 正氣 and immunity in Chinese medicine?

Zhèng qì is that which is innate to the human mind and body, functioning with precision and balance, preventing illness. The *zhèng qì* has the ability to differentiate between "self" and "non-self," the permeability of the skin layer to the external environment, therefore avoiding cold damage, warm disease or wind strike. Immunity is based on the healthy interaction of *yíng qì* and *wèi qì*, and is described in the *Shānghán Lùn* 傷寒論, as three yang and three yin layers of interactivity of the body/mind's correct qi with the outside environment.

6. What is *xié qì* 邪氣/evil qi?

Xié qì can be external, when the seasonal/climatic qi is overwhelming the *zhèng qì* of a human being, or when the *yíng/wèi* dynamic is disturbed, or weakened. In the *Nán Jīng*, there are also internal evils generated by emotions in excess that disturb the internal dynamic via five phase dynamics, including internal wind.

7. What is the role of *zhèng qì* 正氣 and *xié qì* 邪氣 in autoimmune disorders?

Zhèng qì can be strong or weak; evil qi is strong or weak. Once we determine the degree of repletion or vacuity of each, we can calculate the pattern, location, depth, and strength of the illness.

8. How do we measure *bìngyīn* 病因/disease origin in autoimmune disorders?

Using *liù jīng* 六經/six channel theory, we can "reverse engineer" the present illness back to its origins, through understanding constitution, seasonal qi, past traumas, and infections.

9. How do we measure *zhěn hòu* 診後/prognosis in autoimmune disorders?

Through vessel discrimination, tongue diagnosis, abdominal/channel palpation, we can track the future course of illness using six channel, five phase or four aspect theory.

10. What is the role of *yuán qì* 元氣/ source qi in autoimmune disorders?

Source qi can be damaged by environmental toxins, stress, taxation, aging, or repeated contraction of evil qi. *Yuán qì* is like a spring, "the source" of life, and can be eroded over time by these factors.

11. How do we measure *nèishāng* 內傷 in autoimmune disorders?

By taking a complete history of a patient's illnesses, major life events, traumas, and living situation. This is described in detail in *Sùwèn* 76 and 77. Internal damage is also revealed in vessel discrimination (pulse diagnosis), and other diagnostic methods.

12. How do we measure *wàigǎn* 外感 in autoimmune disorders?

The *Shānghán Lùn* and related texts teach the symptom patterns of external contractions, which are then confirmed by vessel discrimination, tongue diagnosis, and palpation.

13. What is the role of *yīng* 應 in autoimmune disorders?

Yīng or resonance, in my interpretation, is the level of harmonious communication between visceral systems, channels, the three burners, *yíng* and *wèi*, and the vital substances.

14. What is the role of *xiāng huǒ* 相火/ ministerial fire in autoimmune disorders?

All defense qi is rooted in ministerial fire and its circulation in *tàiyáng*, expressed as well in the triple burner, gall bladder (*shào yáng* 少陽), and *xīn zhǔ* 心主/pericardium channels, and their dynamics.

15. How do we measure *xiāng huǒ* 相火/ ministerial fire in autoimmune disorders?

We can look for temperature differentials, sensations of hot and cold, *sì nì* 四逆/four extremities cold, strength in the pulse, coloration of the tongue, warm, coolness, muscle tone of the abdomen, and complexion.

III. Ministerial Fire and Autoimmunity in the *Nán Jīng* 難經

In the *Nán Jīng* 難經 3, vessel examination is considered to be divided between yang at the exterior, yin in the interior, yang in the *cùn* 寸/inch position, yin in the *chǐ* 尺/foot position. These are normal locations. When there is counterflow, yang can invade the yin domain, and yin invade the yang domain. This is palpable, and finding yin qi or yang qi in the wrong location means that yin and yang have lost regulation.

In autoimmune disorders, clearly yin and yang qi have lost their mutual interaction and correct placement in the mind and body. *Yíng* and *wèi* lose their regulation, the flow of qi and blood is chaotic, and the breath and heartbeat may become erratic. With *Nán Jīng*-style acupuncture, we apply five phase theory to acupuncture treatment strategies involving the *wǔ shū xué* 五俞穴/five transporting holes to regulate the flow of *yíng* and *wèi*, yin and yang qi. In *Nán Jīng* 難經 3, the *guān* 關/gate is seen as a barrier between the *cùn* 寸/inch and *chǐ* 尺/foot positions. The length of these two positions (long or short), and overflowing or not reaching qualities, determines what the text calls *fù* 覆/turnover or *yì* 益/overflow. *Guān* 關/(external) closure and *gé* 格/barrier, according to Katō Bankei, refers to a disease where *yīn*, located in the *chǐ* 尺 realm, and *yáng*, located in the *cùn* 寸 realm, displace each other. This is an example of *nì* 逆/counterflow, where the correct placement of internal/external, upper and lower, and *yīn* and *yáng* qualities is displaced and moves to circumvent the normal order (of *yīn* and *yáng qì*) of the body.

IV. Qi Transformation and Ministerial Fire in Lǐ Dōngyuán's Spleen Stomach Theory

The *Píwèi Lùn* 脾胃论 has a pivotal statement on which we can focus quite a bit of attention in trying to understand autoimmune disease from a Chinese medical perspective:

> Ministerial fire is the fire of the pericardium developing from the lower burner. It is a foe to the original qi. (This yin) fire and the original qi are irreconcilable to each other. When one is victorious, the other must be the loser.[5]

My explanation of this theory is as follows: the *xiāng huǒ* 相火/ministerial fire, also known as *mìng mén huǒ* 命門火/life gate fire, is the fire of the lower burner, which, according to the *Nàn Jīng* 難經, resides between the two kidneys. One can imagine it as a pilot light, a level flame which maintains the metabolic heat of an organism. If too low, kidney yang vacuity or dual spleen/kidney yang vacuity may develop, leading to a cold and sore lower back and legs, clear, copious urination, and diarrhea with undigested food particles (clear food diarrhea). However, if the ministerial fire is stirred, it rises up, damaging the spleen and stomach and disturbing the heart. The ministerial fire is stimulated by over-exertion, overwork, alcohol, smoking, recreational drugs such as cocaine, prescription drugs such as prednisone, excessive sexual activity, loud music, violent movies, and late-night partying. This excessive stirring of ministerial fire eventually consumes the *yuán qì* 原氣/original qi, which is composed of *dà qì* 大氣/air qi from the lungs combined with *gǔ qì* 穀氣/food qi from the spleen and *jīng* 精/essence from the kidneys to support the organism.[6]

In the *Píwèi Lùn*, Lǐ Dōngyuán describes complex diseases

5   Dongyuan, L. & Flaws, B. (2004) *Li Dong-Yuan's Treatise on the Spleen & Stomach: A Translation of the Pi Wei Lun*. Boulder, CO: Blue Poppy Press, p.82.

6   Rosenberg, Z. (2018) *Returning to the Source: Han Dynasty Medical Classis in Modern Clinical Practice*. London: Singing Dragon, pp.73–74.

that greatly resemble such illnesses as multiple sclerosis, for just one example. These complex conditions developed under adverse conditions in central China during the Jin-Yuan dynasty on the central plains, where war, famine, and stress greatly depleted spleen/stomach qi, with resulting chaos in *yíng/wèi* defenses of the body. Lǐ Dōngyuán observed that the body seemed to be attacking itself, and in his theory described the collapse of defense qi that fell internally, accumulating in the abdomen and causing vacuity heat evils. He called these evils "yin fire." Yin fire, according to Lǐ Dōngyuán, was an accumulation of heat in the middle burner due to the *sān jiāo* 三焦/triple burner not distributing ministerial fire throughout the organism. When the middle burner is vacuous, the upper and lower burners cannot communicate well, and both the up-bearing of yang qi and descent of yin qi are interrupted, leading to chaos, and the inability of the spleen and stomach to separate the clear and turbid qi from food and liquids. Lǐ Dōngyuán states that this yin fire arises from the lower *jiāo* and becomes intertwined with the heart and then loses its governing power, which is when the ministerial fire takes control. He discusses that the ministerial fire is the encircling fire of the lower burner and is the thief of the source qi. In Zhāng Jǐngyuè's critique of this idea, he says that the ministerial fire can never be synonymous with evil qi, that any evil heat in the body will be the result of excesses of emotions that damage the correct qi, not the ministerial fire itself.

V. Causative Factors of Autoimmune Disease

Why are we seeing so many complex autoimmune disorders, from respiratory and digestive allergies to lupus and rheumatoid arthritis? Some of the reasons are outlined below.

Over-treatment with pharmaceutical drugs

Many drugs are immunosuppressive and, especially when several powerful drugs from different classes are combined, this can lead to immune chaos.

Constitutional weaknesses inherited from parents

As environmental, dietary, emotional, and social influences increase over several generations, this is also reflected in the quality of *jīng* 精/essence generated by parents. There is an insidious influence on future generations from in vitro fertilization and fertility drugs, aging new parents, and medical interventions at birth (premature babies, etc.). As parents postpone having children due to career and financial pressures, and damage is caused to the lower burner in women by long-term use of birth control pills (which dampen the ministerial fire necessary for fertility), their bodies' strength declines with age, reducing fertility. Resorting to "artificial *jīng*" may produce success in having children, but at a reduced storage of original *jīng*.

Biàn zhèng 變證/Transmuted patterns

Zhāng Zhòngjǐng emphasized transmuted patterns in the *Shānghán Lùn* 傷寒論, distorted immune responses to illness due to mistreatment or suppression. Unless an illness is treated both root and branch, and resolved by treating each patient individually and with a whole-systems, complexity approach, the illness will often become more complex, stubborn, and deep-rooted.

Qíng shāng 情傷/Emotional damage

Emotional overload is the norm in modern culture, as we are bombarded with constant news events, family dramas, isolation, obsessiveness, and the excesses that a culture alienated from nature will produce.

Láo Sǔn 劳损/*Taxation detriment*

Chinese medical texts define several types of taxation: work taxation, bedroom taxation, emotional taxation, and food taxation among them. Taxation interferes with the normal, rhythmic interchange of yin and yang, eventually leading to *juéyīn* disorder. Yin and yang then separate, ministerial fire floats to the upper burner, harassing the heart and lungs, while the lower burner is cold and vacuous.

The assault on normal nutrition by "food-like substances," pesticides, bioengineering and extreme counteracting "diets"

As the soil loses its essences, through over-cultivation, mono-cropping, hybridization, and genetically modified products, both vegetable and animal foods become weakened in vitality and nutrition. The over-processed "foods," loaded with preservatives to increase shelf life, fill people with empty calories and with little nutrition, leading to obesity and diabetes epidemics. Often, people are led to try extreme diets to balance out all of the excess and fool their metabolisms into losing (or gaining) weight, which leads to further illness and complex disorders.

Environmental factors

These include air, water, soil pollution, pesticides, heavy metals, and food additives. As discussed previously in this book, we have reached a "critical mass" of pollutants, with micro-particles of plastic being found at high altitudes, and thousands of forever chemicals permanently embedded in the landscape. Like a human patient overwhelmed by medications and recreational drugs, the oceans, atmosphere, and soil have been compromised in their ability to transmute and detoxify waste materials.

Modern medicine attempts to put out the fire with steroids, antibiotics, and anti-inflammatories, but this is only masking the underlying patho-dynamics. The complex, sophisticated model of immunology is an engineering model, based on mechanisms that are then treated with medications designed to modify these mechanisms in such a way that symptoms are reduced or suppressed. In biomedicine, cytokines are seen as a cause of inflammation associated with aging. Chronic, systematic inflammation is seen to cause organ damage and a range of diseases from autoimmune disorders to cancer. If we make the mistake of seeing this inflammation as "evil heat" or "yin vacuity," we will often make the wrong therapeutic decisions for our patients. Many modern Chinese medicine practitioners end up giving cold, bitter, draining formulas or heavy, greasy yin supplementing formulas with the idea that the "steroidal, anti-inflammatory effect" mimics biomedical approaches, either consciously or unconsciously.

We can understand one aspect of zhèng qì 正氣/correct qi as the weakening of healthy microbiomes from poor diet, and the overuse of pharmaceuticals. The overuse of medications leads to the disturbance of microflora environments in the stomach and large intestine, allowing xié qì 邪氣, destructive microorganisms, viruses, bacteria, mold, fungi, and yeast to proliferate.

The inflammation of joints, tissues, and organs, along with fevers, sweating, and body aches, is indicative of the disharmony of yíng qì 營氣 and wèi qì 衛氣, and the ministerial fire attempting to unblock channels, blood, and fluid circulation, mainly through the shàoyáng 少陽 and juéyīn 厥陰 channel pathways. Cold often will accumulate, or alternate with heat (as is common in shàoyáng and juéyīn disease), and the ministerial fire attempts to warm the cold accumulations, but often will get "stuck" in articulations and joints, or will inflame tissues. I've read a few Chinese medicine textbooks,[7] which tend to mimic biomedical treatments and include "anti-inflammatory herbs," according to biomedical definition, which tend to be bitter and cold. One textbook relies on *wēn bìng xué* 温病学/warm disease theory, and frames autoimmune disorders as acute warm diseases, which is highly unlikely, as the "incubation" period is long and gradual, unlike epidemic diseases. There is a lot of emphasis on supplementing yin, and many Chinese medicine herbalists try to employ herbs for their "steroidal" effect. Attacking acute symptoms with large doses of bitter cold herbs in large formulas may damage spleen qi, aggravating an underlying depletion of ministerial fire. Supplementing yin with heavy, greasy herbs such as *shú dì huáng* 熟地黄/rehmanniae radix praeparata may congest the middle burner and lead to stickiness and obstruction in the lower burner.

VI. Ecological Medicine and Autoimmune Disorders

Classically, Chinese medicine has treated all health issues as a disconnect between heaven, earth, and human life. *Sùwèn* 素問 3, which is translated as *Comprehensive Discourse on Regulating the Spirit in Accordance with the Qi of the Four Seasons*, emphasizes living in accordance with each season, adapting to weather and climatic changes, addressing diet, activity, clothing, emotions, and sleep. If seasonal qi is chaotic, this leads to damage to crops, and animal and human health.

Our disconnect from nature, the progressive development of enslaving all natural elements and kingdoms to provide for human

---

7   See Hou, W. (2011) *Treating Autoimmune Disease with Chinese Medicine.* London: Churchill Livingstone Press.

need and pleasure, has led to an unsustainable consumption of resources and the alarming disappearance of untold species. The artificial life support structures we have enabled to be able to live in otherwise adverse environments (transporting water to deserts, tapping underground aquifers, draining swamps, cutting down forests, paving over land with concrete, installing air conditioning and central heating, building skyscrapers with no open windows from synthetic materials, using artificial lighting) have led to this disconnect between humanity and the rest of creation. "Sick building syndrome" is just one example of how our health has been impacted from this, and the COVID-19 pandemic is an example of a scourge that took advantage of these conditions. I highly recommend reading my first book, *Returning to the Source*, which makes the argument in detail as to how and why Chinese medicine is ecological medicine. It explains that humanity is part of an ecological continuum, which the Han dynasty physicians believed was the interface between heaven and earth and how we as humans had great power to influence our planet, but the side effects of our technologies have led to the consumption of the yin aspect of earth. Just as our environment changes, so does the environment of our bodies. Moises Velasquez-Manoff writes in his book, *An Epidemic of Absence*:

> To treat modernity's ailments, consider not only the human genome, but also our meta-genome; the other 99 percent of instructions necessary to smoothly operate the human super-organism. And rather than clear-cut, actively cultivate. Germ theory has brought us a long way. But in order to continue maximizing our health and well-being, and that of our loved ones, we've got to eschew the brute-force tactics of the exterminator, adopt the gardener's finesse, and grow the super organism.[8]

8   Velasques-Manoff, M. (2013) *An Epidemic of Absence: A New Way of Understanding Allergies and Autoimmune Diseases*. New York, NY: Scribner, p.307.

In losing contact with what he calls the ecosystem's "superorganism," that is, the soil and its natural microorganisms, we harm our immune systems, which leads to allergies and other autoimmune disorders.

One of the antidotes for the environmental degradation I mention above is the fungi family, specifically the myriads of mushroom species that populate the planet. Many of these, of course, are used in Chinese medicine and by native populations around the planet. Many mushrooms are being researched for their ability to neutralize plastic, carbon, and chemical pollution, even radiation in nuclear power plants. The present epidemic has woken up many to how alienated humanity has become from the essential factors that nurture and support life. Modern biomedicine and naturopathic medicine have discovered the microbiome, which connects the health of our internal environment with the external one, and a healthy microbiome is like healthy soil, teeming with life and microorganisms.

CHAPTER 7

MINISTERIAL FIRE AND MENOPAUSE

Hot Flashes are *Not* Necessarily Yin Vacuity

A common mistake in modern Chinese medicine circles is to consider menopausal hot flashes and night sweats to be solely kidney yin vacuity, causing deficient yin heat to rise upwards. Formulas such as *zhī bǎi dì huáng wán* 知柏地黄丸/anemarrhena, phellodendron, and rehmannia pill and *liù wèi dì huáng wán* 六味地黄丸/six ingredient pill with rehmannia, are chosen to strongly supplement yin and/or descend fire with cold bitter substances. However, patients with kidney yin vacuity need to show the following signs:

- heat in the palms and soles of feet

- a shriveled, cracked red tongue, often mirror-like

- a rapid, thready pulse

- sore throat, teeth and gums

- lower back soreness and pain

- prolonged low-grade fever

- disturbed sleep with intense dreaming.

Then formulas such as the above or formulas such as Lǐ Dōngyuán 李東垣's *dāng guī liù huáng tāng* 當歸六黃湯/tangkuei and six yellow decoction can be used, and will be very successful. This formula combines *dāng guī* 當歸/angelicae sinensis radix to nourish blood, *huáng qí*/astragali radix to raise clear yang, dried and prepared rehmannia (*shú dì huáng* 熟地黃/rehmanniae radix praeparata) to strongly nourish yin, and the "three *huáng*" (*huáng qín* 黃芩/scutellariae radix, *huáng lián* 黃連/coptidis rhizoma and *huáng bǎi* 黃柏/phellodendri cortex) to descend fire.

Yin vacuity in menopause became a popular diagnosis as the result of the influence of biomedical ideas on Chinese medicine in the 1960s, when hormone replacement therapy became used on a wide scale to control menopausal symptoms. Chinese medicine doctors astutely observed that hormones such as estrogen had a heavy, dense, cold nature, and a *jīng* 精-like quality. They also observed that in formulas such as *liù wèi dì huáng wán*/six ingredient pill with rehmannia, that the herb *shānyào* 山藥/dioscoreae rhizome was a source of phytoestrogens, and that the dioscorea family (dioscorea mexicana) was the original source for synthesizing birth control pills.[1]

The theories of Zhū Dānxī 朱丹溪 outlined in *Dān Xī Xīn Fǎ* 丹溪心法/*Heart Method of Dānxī* state that "yang is always abundant and the yin always insufficient." This concept became very popular in the mid-20th century, as it seemed to fit many of these vacuity fire conditions. However, his *zī yīn pài* 滋陰派/nourish the yin current, was largely discredited even in his own era as eccentric and not consistent with classical theory![2] Ministerial fire, or dragon

---

1   See the autobiography, Djerassi, C. (1992) *The Pill, Pygmy Chimps, and Degas' Horse: The Remarkable Autobiography of the Award-winning Scientist who Synthesized the Birth-Control Pill.* New York, NY: Basic Books, for a description of how biochemist Carl Djerassi first synthesized the birth control pill from dioscorea mexicana.

2   See the writings of Zhāng Jingyuè and Ekiken Kaibara, who strongly dispute Zhū Dānxī 's positions on ministerial fire and supplementing yin.

fire, is the fire that resides in water, and is in its correct relationship when it remains "submerged." If water becomes superabundant in the lower burner, and the ministerial fire is weakened, the fire will be displaced and "float" towards the upper burner.

If one diagnoses many menopausal women correctly, one will often find that they have pale swollen tongues with red tips, and cold soft bellies, clear urination, poor digestion, and fatigue. This indicates lower burner yang vacuity with ministerial fire flaring upwards. The key is to supplement kidney yang and/or descend the floating fire by warming the lower burner. The original kidney supplementing formula, *shèn qì wán* 腎氣丸/kidney qi pill, is superior to *liù wèi dì huáng wán*/six ingredient pill with rehmannia, which was originally designed by Qián Yǐ 錢乙 in the 12th century as a pediatric formula for small children with weak constitutions and yin substance, for the *wǔ chí* 五遲/five retardations,[3] and *shèn qiè* 腎怯/kidney timidity. By removing the yang supplementing ingredients (*fù zǐ* 附子/aconiti radix lateralis and *guì zhī* 桂枝/cinnamomi ramulus), and adding *shú dì huáng* 熟地黃/rehmanniae radix praeparata, this formula becomes a cooler, heavier formula with very different indications.

As with all other systematic issues, we first need to understand the root cause of the ascending fire, the specific channels, and affected *zàng fǔ* 臟腑, and then treat accordingly. There are many formulas used in Chinese medicine for menopausal issues. One is *wēn jīng tāng* 溫經湯/warm the flow decoction, which includes *wú zhū yú* 吳茱萸/evodiae fructus that has a strong descending action and brings the ministerial fire back to its source in the lower burner. I find this formula especially useful when the *chōng* 衝 and *rèn* 任 channels are not regulated, and the menstrual flow is becoming erratic. Sometimes we need to directly warm the lower burner with a *fù zǐ*/aconiti radix lateralis formula, such as *zhēn*

---

3   Delays in standing, walking, hair growth, tooth eruption/growth and speaking.

wǔ tāng 真武湯/true warrior decoction. Sometimes we need to unblock blood stasis in the lower burner while warming the yang. A formula combination Suzanne Robidoux shared with me that I find effective from Hú Xīshù 胡希恕's *jīng fāng* 經方 school is *dāng guī sháo yào sǎn* 當歸芍藥散/angelica and peony powder combined with *guì zhī fú líng wán* 桂枝茯苓丸/cinnamon twig and poria pill.

In conclusion, we should always examine our thinking in the realm of diagnosis and treatment, and be sure that we are actually using Chinese medical principles rather than those superimposed from biomedicine. Otherwise, we will be prone to clinical errors that could be avoided.

CHAPTER 8

BIÀN ZHĒNG 變蒸/STEAMING AND TRANSFORMATIONS IN NEONATES

Z'ev Rosenberg and Stephen Cowan

(Inspired by Sabine Wilm's translation of the *xiǎo'érkē* 小儿科/pediatrics section of *Bèi Jí Qiānjīn Yào Fāng* 備急千金要方.)

Z'ev: As translated by Sabine Wilms in *Venerating the Root Part I*, Sūn Sīmiǎo 孫思邈 writes in his magnum opus, *Bèi Jí Qiānjīn Yào Fāng* 備急千金要方, about *biàn zhēng* 變蒸/steaming and transformations in neonates as various stages of development.[1] What we can learn from his writing is, first of all, that a Chinese medical physician needs to recognize these normal, but sometimes dramatic transformations as different from exterior evils attacking the defense qi at the exterior. Dr. Sūn points out that the ears and buttocks remain cool in transformations, but are reddened and warm in *shānghán* 傷寒 conditions.

The timing in child rearing and treatment is of extreme importance. Because of the flourishing of yang qi, conditions change quickly and dramatically. A simple wind strike, cold damage, or

---

1   See Wilms, S. (2013) *Venerating the Root Part I*. Corbett, OR: Happy Goat Productions, pp.14–45.

warm disease can quickly penetrate to the yin layers of the body. If the right treatment is given, anything from cool compresses made with tofu or apple juice to warm baths, shonishin 小兒鍼,[2] guā shā 刮痧, gentle needling, and herbal medicine can turn around these conditions quickly. But if not caught in time, there can be great harm, Hashem forbid.

Stephen: Children are strong yang within yin. The spirit is seen as being yang entering the *Shēn tǐ* 身体 body, which is immature yin. *Lǎozǐ* 老子 55 states that an infant's unwitting virtue (*dé* 德) manifests at the maximum limits of *jīng* 精 and harmony (*hé* 和) and this closely resembles the unfinished open-ended state of the Dao Process. An infant is existentially living at such a maximum state of "becoming," physically, cognitively, and spiritually integrated. Dr. Sūn seems to deeply respect this tenuous state of developmental yang heat necessary to produce the sequential stages of growth and cautions us to avoid unnecessarily treating this as pathological heat unless it goes on for too long a period of time or with overly intense flaring heat. I can't help but wonder whether Dr. Sūn was sensing the evidence of ministerial fire at work here as the engine of infant development. I am also keenly aware that the specific timing of these "steamings," which Dr. Sūn mapped out for us, occur at the very same ages that conventional pediatrics recommends vaccinating children (2, 4, 6, 12, 15, and 18 months). I have personally seen this result in added burden of inflammation, which in some children can result in prolonged states of latent heat. Furthermore, this developmental yang heat when replete must discharge in order to allow growth to continue, according to Dr. Sūn. If we suppress this process with too much "cooling down" (e.g. early introduction of over-processed baby formulas and other "cold" foods, the common overuse of antipyretics

---

2   The Japanese rendering of the term er zhēn 兒鍼 meaning child needle

in conventional pediatrics practices, as well as the excessive use of antibiotics and steroids, which are bitter and cold), we run the risk of altering the natural functions of *sān jiāo* 三焦 and ministerial fire. Rapid growth and transformation leads to repletion heat events. Symptoms such as flushed cheeks, fever, reddened eyes, thick mucous, hot, or smelly diarrhea that is green or yellow may appear during steamings. But after steamings are complete, the eyes become noticeably clear.

A baby's life cycle begins with the foundation of ministerial fire rooted in a yin body. It takes time for this yang aspect of spirit to take root in the yin, and there are stages of development discussed in such pediatric texts as the *Bèi Jí Qiānjīn Yào Fāng* section on *xiǎo'érkē* 小儿科/pediatrics. As the process of cellular division and growth continues (it begins from the moment of conception, the meeting of yin and yang), the yang transformations of *shēn tǐ* 身體/body, qi and blood are dramatic and powerful. This process continues after the baby is born to the world and leaves its womb space. As the baby matures, yang qi will sometimes "spill over" and create heat, visible in agitation and excessive movement. In mild cases, we see heat with fright, cold ears and buttocks, slight sweating and white blisters on the upper lip and head. If serious, there may be a chaotic pulse, decreased appetite, vomiting up of milk, slight redness in the whites of the eyes and slight whiteness in the black of the eyes.[3]

Z'ev: In paediatrics, we diagnose exterior evils/*shānghán* 傷寒 by rubbing the index finger to raise a vein, which is divided into wind, qi, and blood aspects, and palpating the abdomen and gently touching head, limbs, buttocks, and ears. In Tibetan medicine, one can diagnose exterior evils by examining the back of the ears, looking for visible blood vessels in the upper, middle, and lower

---

3   Ibid., p.17.

part of the ear. I myself use this method in my practice, and find it to be highly effective. As the child grows, the *cùn kǒu* 寸口 pulse becomes more complex and differentiated, and the physician can move from using one finger to two fingers/positions after age three, and all three fingers by age 12, when a full pulse diagnosis is possible. In small children, the tongue is a very reliable method of reading the interior condition, and often the changes in the tongue are very dramatic during external attacks.

If exterior attacks do occur, they will often lead to the expelling of what Chinese medicine calls *tāidú* 胎毒/fetal toxin, boils, or skin eruptions, a combination of wind and interior evil heat generated in the womb. Many childhood illnesses such as measles, mumps, and chickenpox fall into this category, as do strong febrile conditions with rashes such as roseola, and must be managed carefully by the physician. In all cases, it is necessary to discriminate between steaming/transformation cycles and fetal toxin combined with evil qi. As with steaming and transformation, these febrile illnesses are often followed by growth spurts and new stages of development.

Stephen: *Lǎozǐ* 55 recommends that we look to the infant to behold the embodied manifestation of virtue (*dé* 德). Sūn Sīmiǎo's profound observation that there are discreetly timed "steamings" (*zhēng* 蒸) that drive growth and transformation (*biàn* 變) in children provides a subtle but critically important differentiation between physiologic warmth and pathologic heat. This physiologic warmth in young children is objective evidence of ministerial fire's action, facilitating *yuán qì* 元氣's function of supporting growth and development through the *sān jiāo* 三焦. Unfortunately in our modern western medicine, this has been all but ignored; we suppress every sign of heat with antipyretics (tylenol damaging the liver/glutathione production), and the proscribed timing of vaccinations in early childhood falls exactly when Sūn Sīmiǎo tells us that the steamings take place, thus adding additional heat to an already taxed biologic system.

Qián Yǐ 錢乙, the great Song dynasty pediatrician, was acutely aware of the difference between physiologic steaming and pathologic heat in his herbal innovations. His transformation of Zhāng Zhòngjǐng 張仲景's *bā wèi dì huáng tang* 八味地黃湯 into *liù wèi dì huáng wán* 六味地黃丸/six ingredient pill with rehmannia, for use in young children to support growth and development, was particularly important. He recognized that children during intense developing stages of the first years of life require a milder, gentler form of support, removing *fù zǐ* 附子/aconiti radix lateralis and *ròu guì* 肉桂/cinnamomi cortex in order to avoid overstimulating the already yang-prone state.

Z'ev: It is ironic that *liù wèi dì huáng wán* has become much more widely used in modern Chinese medicine practice, well beyond the original indications in pediatrics for developmental issues. Qián Yǐ recognized that children's yang qi is fulminant and highly active... and reactive! But for elderly people, supplementing yin without yang will only lead to reduced spleen qi transformation, cold and damp accumulating in the abdomen, and a massive waste of beneficial herbal ingredients.

Stephen: Lǐ Dōngyuán 李東垣, applauded Qián Yǐ's approach, recognizing the importance of dietary therapy in supporting the spleen–stomach balance with more neutral foods like rice congee so that this engendering and transforming does not expire. Master Lǐ further noted the importance of dietary and medicinal adaptations to the four seasons, thus giving us a picture of our own health reflecting the health of the planet and our dependence on harmonizing with environmental forces. In the *Píwèi Lùn* 脾胃論, he writes:

the *Nèijīng* 內經 [states that the treatment] must anticipate the yearly qi [i.e. weather changes particular to a certain year] and avoid infringing on the heavenly harmony [or natural laws of weather in the four seasons] to be a consummate treatment.[4]

As a pediatrician, I am continually confronted with the epidemic of "too much too fast" in our culture, manifesting in body-mind-spirit reactions to excess overstimulation coupled with a lack of yin nourishment. The foundation of Chinese medicine (the *Yìjīng* 易經) recognizes the delicate balance needed to deal with change. Our western culture is obsessed with never-ending growth, excitement, and convenience that disconnects us from the natural cycles of the planet we evolved to thrive on. The flipside of this obsession is an utter intolerance of boredom, frustration, and discomfort. Climate change is a profound manifestation of this disconnection. It is no wonder that we are seeing epidemics of allergies, autism, ADHD, autoimmune disease, and Alzheimer's in our culture.

---

4   Dongyuan, L. & Flaws, B. (2004) *Li Dong-Yuan's Treatise on the Spleen & Stomach: A Translation of the Pi Wei Lun.* Boulder, CO: Blue Poppy Press, p.292.

Biàn Zhēng 變蒸/Steaming & Transformations in Neonates

- After steaming, eyes become clear
- Rapid growth and transformation leads to relation heat events
- Timing in child raising and treatment of extreme importance
- Physician needs to recognize normal transformation from exterior evils attacking
- Yang spirit enters yin *shēn tǐ* 身体 body
- Children are strong yang within yin
- Effect of vaccines, antibiotics and steroids upon emerging yang qi
- Ears and buttock are cool in transformation and warm in *shānghán* 傷寒 conditions

Steaming & Transformations in Neonates

CHAPTER 9

CASE STUDIES

What is different about the case studies in this book from the first two books in this series is that I use the same or similar formulas in all three cases, in order to illustrate how "same formula, different disease" may work, especially with a specific subject such as ministerial fire. But by no means am I suggesting limiting one's formula repertoire to just a handful of formulas.

Case Study 1

In late October 2008, a 49-year-old male complained of erectile dysfunction. He complained that his penis felt numb and cold. He also had occasional nausea, vomiting, and dizziness, and suffered from constant fatigue. His pulse was a bit rapid (he was a regular coffee drinker, not surprising given his continual lack of energy). The pulse was thin and vacuous, specifically in the chi positions (right and left kidney) and *cùn* 寸 positions (hand *shàoyīn* 少陰 and hand *tàiyīn* 太陰). The tongue showed some heat signs, with a thin yellow coating.

This patient was a student at an acupuncture college who I used to see in the clinic, and he practiced an intensive form of qi gong along with weightlifting and running. I warned him then, several years before, that his low back pain, cold penis, seminal emission, vertigo, and extreme fatigue were signs of depletion of the ministerial fire stored in the kidney. At the time, I treated him, with some success, with *guì zhī jiā lóng gǔ mǔ lì tāng* 桂枝加龍骨牡蠣湯/cinnamon twig decoction plus dragon bone and oyster shell, but he failed to completely refrain from his extreme activity. Several years later, although he had children with his wife, many of his symptoms still remained.

I then treated him first with a raw formula (see below), which is a modification of *bǔ zhōng yì qì tāng* 補中益氣湯/tonify the middle to augment the qi decoction, plus medicinals to supplement kidney yang. I later solidified treatment with prepared extracts of *bǔ zhōng yì qì tāng*/tonify the middle to augment the qi decoction, and *shèn qì wán* 腎氣丸/kidney qi pill. I also prescribed for him a liquid extract of *dōng chóng xià cǎo* 冬蟲夏草/cordyceps, to strengthen his kidneys, and recommended a diet of only warming foods, such as soups, ginger, garlic and lots of whole grains, wild salmon, miso soup, and vegetables. He did not want acupuncture at this point, so I told him which points to moxa at home, specifically Ren 4–6, KI 16, ST 36, and back shu points such as BL 23, 28, and 38, with the help of his wife.

> *huáng qí* 黃芪/astragali radix 18–24g
> *rén shēn* 人参/ginseng radix 12g
> *bái zhú* 白朮/atractylodis macrocephalae rhizoma 9g
> *zhì gān cǎo* 炙甘草/glycyrrhizae radix praeparata 6g
> *chénpí* 陈皮/citri reticulate pericarpium 4.5g
> *bàn xià* 半夏/pinelliae rhizoma praeparata 9g
> *chái hú* 柴胡/bupleuri radix 9g
> *guì zhī* 桂枝/cinnamomi ramulus 6g
> *dāng gui* 当归/angelicae sinensis radix 9g
> *chuān xiōng* 川芎/chuanxiong rhizoma 4.5g
> *shú dì huáng* 熟地黃/rehmanniae radix praeparata 9g
> *dù zhòng* 杜仲/eucommiae cortex 9g
> *wǔ wèi zǐ* 五味子/schisandrae fructus 6g

gǒu qǐ zǐ 枸杞子/lycii fructus 6g
shān zhū yú 山茱萸/corni fructus 4.5g
fú líng 茯苓/poria 6g

He stopped coming, as he lived out in the desert many miles from my office. After many years, I saw this patient again (2021), and aging had only increased his problems. He passed kidney stones every few months, and had retired from his acupuncture and *tai na* massage practice. His diet was not good, and he had rib pain on the right side, what he described as gall bladder symptoms, occasional arrhythmias, constant diarrhea, a detached retina, floaters, and poor vision. His pulse now had a spike in the right *cùn* position, a soggy deep right *guān* 關 (*tàiyīn* spleen vacuity), and a spike in the right *chǐ* 尺 position, connected most likely with his kidney stones. His left-hand pulse had a spike in the left *cùn* position, a deep *guān*, vacuous with a wiry core, and a depleted *chǐ* pulse. His tongue was now pale, purple, and tender, showing severe inner cold.

My diagnosis was a *shàoyīn* 少陰 water/fire imbalance with depleted ministerial fire, middle burner depletion with wood/earth imbalance, with ministerial fire rising up on occasion to disturb his heart qi and lung qi, leading to overall *tàiyīn* qi vacuity. I gave him a liquid extract combining *shèn qì wán* 腎氣丸/kidney qi pill, *tiān xióng sàn* 天雄散/tianxiong aconite powder, and *zhēn wǔ tāng* 真武湯/true warrior decoction, one third each to warm and supplement ministerial fire, and enhance kidney and sexual function.

On his next visit, two weeks later, he allowed me to treat him with acupuncture and moxibustion. He was constantly fatigued, not sleeping well, and busy doing construction work (which seemed inappropriate given his age and condition). He mentioned suffering from depression and anxiety, an inability to make decisions (gall bladder/ministerial fire issues), and added a weak urinary stream and enlarged prostate to the symptoms. I added cannabidiol (CBD) oil to help him with sleep, and encouraged him to continue the herbs long term, including the cordyceps extract. I applied moxa to KI 1. GB 21, Du 15, BL 11, 14, and 23 were needled with moxa on BL 23. On the front, I treated unilaterally opposite sides KI 2 with HT 3, LI 5 with ST 41, plus KI 16 with moxa, Ren 5 with moxa, LR 14 and KI 27.

He has not followed up with me since June, but recently notified me that he is ready to again do treatment.

Case Study 2

In late November 2020, a 50-year-old male contracted COVID-19 from his girlfriend. He complained of bone, muscle, and nerve pain, along with fever and chills, occipital headache, and a loss of appetite. He developed a dry cough, and what felt like lung congestion. He was treated by his homeopath with the remedy eupatorium.[1] It took two weeks for him to begin to feel better. On our Zoom consult, he noted that he still had fatigue that came and went, with no shortness of breath. His tongue was short and stiff with a red tip. Eating grains or beans seemed to increase the fatigue, which indicated that his spleen qi was still weak. His sleep was interrupted and not restful. I suggested he find a local acupuncturist to treat him once or twice a week, and had him moxa his abdominal area in a circle around the navel. I recommended two formulas: the first was *chái hú guì zhī tāng* 柴胡桂枝湯/bupleurum and cinnamon twig decoction to harmonize the *wèi qì* 衛氣 and *yíng qì* 營氣, harmonize the stomach, and resolve any *shàoyáng* 少陽 pathogens, followed up after one week with *bǔ zhōng yì qì tāng*/tonify the middle to augment the qi decoction, to strengthen spleen qi, and raise the clear yang.

---

[1]   A genus of flowering plants in the aster family, *pèi lán* 佩蘭.

We met again six months later (May 2021), with a post-COVID syndrome presentation. His sleep patterns were erratic, and he was waking about 3–4am. His symptoms were cyclical he was getting waves of fatigue, pressure headaches, and distinct pressure in his ears. He had cardiac symptoms that began six weeks earlier— chest pain with radiating sensations, and feeling as if he was going to faint or collapse. An electrocardiogram and other tests found no heart damage. He normally tended to low blood pressure. He also presented with low back pain and a weak urinary stream. This time, the tongue was pale, with a dark tip and toothmarks. My diagnosis and observation was as follows:

The COVID-19 invasion, as for many sufferers, devastated his yang qi as the *wèi qì* and *yíng qì* at the *tàiyáng* 太陽 aspect attempted to protect the interior yin domain from damage. Infections such as these are greatly influenced by seasonal qi, which was moving rapidly into a very yin state (one month before winter solstice), by colder weather, and by living at high altitude in very dry air. What is not always recognized by Chinese medicine practitioners is that even in exterior invasions that have a strong heat aspect, such as *yángmíng* 陽明 channel, combination *yángmíng* 陽明/*shàoyáng* 少陽 disease, or qi aspect disorders (in warm disease pattern differentiation) may consume the ministerial fire. The ministerial fire bolsters all qi transformations, and attempts to expel evil qi through the exterior by thrusting out from interior yin to exterior yang. If there is excessive sweating, heat effusion/fever or chill, the ministerial fire will be depleted. In extreme scenarios, such as COVID-19, this can allow the pathogen to sink inwards and impact the yin/internal viscera. The exterior of the body is governed by *tàiyáng*, but is bolstered and supported by *shàoyīn* 少陰 qi of heart and kidney. If the *shàoyīn* is exhausted, pathogens can easily invade the interior and settle in the heart or kidney, leading to continued fatigue, shortness of breath, irregular heartbeat, rapid heartbeat on exertion (as in postural tachycardia syndrome, or

POTS), weak urination, generalized cold with vexation, cold hands and feet, and/or foggy thinking or "Covid brain."

I suggested another moxa regimen, plus daily gentle qi gong and breathing exercises. The herbal formula I recommended was a combination of *dāng guī sì nì jiā wú zhū yú shēng jiāng tang* 當歸四逆加吳茱萸生薑湯/angelica counterflow cold decoction plus evodia and fresh ginger 50 percent, plus *zhēn wǔ tāng*/true warrior decoction.

Towards the end of July, the patient reported unusual fatigue, that varied day to day. The smoke from recent forest fires in the mountains was bothering him. He tended to feel fine for two weeks, then post-COVID symptoms would come back, with significant fatigue, so he needed to nap an hour, then it lifted. He had burning sensations at LI 11, back of thighs, and the upper shoulders, along the bladder, large intestine, and triple burner channels, specifically *tàiyáng* 太陽. As well as body aches and temporal headaches, he also had pain around the kidney area, and around the *dài mài* 帶脈/belt channel. Sleep was better. Heart rhythms had improved. His tongue had red edges and tip, the body was stiff, and it was thickly coated with red spots. I prescribed *chái hú guì zhī tang* 柴胡桂枝湯/bupleurum and cinnamon twig decoction for one month, then a return to the original formula.

Case Study 3

11/3/2021: patient was a 63-year-old male, diagnosed in 1996 with multiple sclerosis. He was treated with copaxone and betaserone, which made him feel horrible.

He went into a steady decline, to the point where he couldn't write with his right hand, and was limping with weakness in his right leg. Around 8pm, he would get intense pain in his left thigh and arm. He got great results from acupuncture, and went several times a week for several years and began doing qi gong in the mornings in a nearby park. He also suffered from loss of balance. In second grade, he remembered having a, serious "mysterious illness" that changed his personality, making him more withdrawn. He also suffered with deep-seated fear and anxiety, which only recently tapered off at 60 years of age. The patient meditated twice a day, and only had occasional minor twinges of pain or symptoms. His digestion was good, but paradoxically he craved junk food. He was not using any medication, and had not seen a "western" doctor in many years. He retired from work in 1996 when the symptoms first appeared. He used to have difficulty falling asleep. He had sexual function issues (common with MS), softness, and poor erection. He never suffered from flus or colds. He had had a slight slur in his speech in the past, but his speech seemed very clear. His tongue was very pale, with poor tone ("floppy"), and his pulse was deep thin, weak, and rough in all positions.

I diagnosed him with foot *shàoyīn* 少陰 vacuity cold/yang pattern, with weak ministerial fire. I treated him with acupuncture on a bi-weekly basis, utilizing the *yáng qiāo mài* 陽蹻脈 to regulate sleep (SI 3/BL 62) and the *chōng mài* 衝脈 to generate and circulate blood (SP 4/PC 6). I noted that both channels penetrated the brain and benefited the central nervous system. I also needled ST 28 with needle moxa, and KI 9 with moxa and other points. His herbal formulas were *zhēn wǔ tāng*/true warrior decoction and *dāng guī sì nì jiā lóng gǔ mǔ lì tāng* 當歸四逆加吳茱萸生薑湯/angelica counterflow cold decoction plus dragon bone and oyster shell.

Having seen several patients diagnosed with multiple sclerosis over the years, I was astounded at how well this individual seemed to be doing. He seemed very motivated spiritually and was doing a lot of dream work on his own. When I first started my practice, there was a wave of MS cases in the Denver/Boulder area of Colorado, often attributed to the effects of the altitude and sometimes extreme weather changes. But there are also emotional and physical factors, constitutional factors, and the issue of environmental toxins that have become more and more pervasive. Many MS patients have weakened constitutions, and cases may be seen where the parents have less than ideal *jīng* 精/ essence to share with their children, especially if they are in poor health, older, or not taking care of themselves. This, then is in the realm of *jīng*/essence and yang vacuity, which this book discusses further in Appendix II in terms of young children being exposed to cold food and drink, excessive vaccines, and medications. Many of these children will develop autoimmune disorders later in life, specifically after the onset of puberty both in males and females.

In this case study, the patient had done a marvelous job of maintaining his health. But the thin weak pulse and pale floppy tongue indicated that there was still depletion of the ministerial fire and kidney yang. Specifically with acupuncture/moxibustion treatment, it was essential that light stimulus, few needles, and a lot of moxa should be used, as overstimulating the channels would just weaken the patient.

CHAPTER 10

CONCLUSION

21st-Century Ministerial Fire:
From Fossil Fuels to the Sun

The great historical medical sages of China had their interpretations and applications of ministerial and sovereign fire. We have seen, particularly, that *mìng mén* 命門/dragon fire and ministerial fire have been fluid in their meaning through different dynasties/ eras, with their political intrigues, and changes in climate patterns. Each of the great physicians (*dà jiā* 大家) had the task of adapting these teachings to the medical matters of their era. For what is such an essential medical principle, ministerial fire inspired a multitude of positions and perspectives over time.[1]

In *Afterglow*, we have discussed the relationship of yin fire, yang fire, and their essential importance to ecological health, and tied that to human health in an attempt to understand ministerial fire in a less conceptual manner. As our civilization shifts from fossil fuels to solar, wind, water, and other renewable sources of energy, understanding the role of ministerial fire in human health will also become a central concern of Chinese medicine

---

[1] See Chapter 4 on The Picasso Principle in my first book, *Returning to the Source* (Singing Dragon, 2018), where I discuss how a practitioner of Chinese medicine can entertain multiple perspectives in pattern differentiation when diagnosing and treating patients. In the same sense, at this point in time we can examine, critique, and entertain multiple perspectives on phenomena such as ministerial fire.

and healthcare in general. The concept of ministerial fire will become a central pillar not only of Chinese medicine, but world medicine. Since the life force of the human being reflects our own internal sun, managing this life force is one of the essential keys to health. Specifically, qi transformation is powered by ministerial fire, and the abdominal cauldron transforming food and liquids into *qì* 氣, *xuè* 血, and *yíng* 營 depends on this fire. One's immunity to weather changes, seasonal qi, and climate, along with specific pathogens, depends on *wèi qì* 衛氣/defense qi, which is the warmth that covers the membrane surface of our body, and arises from grain qi. The extraction of essential substances, and the separation of the clear and turbid qi, depends on ministerial fire (*xiàng huǒ* 相火). Without ministerial fire, sovereign fire (*jūn huǒ* 君火), the illumination of the heart cannot occur, so our very consciousness depends on this fire circulating freely in *shàoyáng* 少陽/gall bladder and triple burner tracts.

The *huǒ shén pài* 火神派/fire spirit school particularly has lessons for us on stoking our inner fires with "hot coals" from *fù zǐ* 附子/aconiti radix lateralis, *gān jiāng* 乾薑/zingiberis rhizome, and *ròu guì* 肉桂/cinnamomi cortex. Our very immunity, our ability to adapt to changes, depends on this fire, and on restoring the balance of *wèi qì* and *yíng qì* 營氣, yang and yin, exterior and interior, resolving and repairing autoimmunity, which is the chronic illness of our age. When acute illnesses are suppressed through toxic medications, cold herbs and supplements, poor diet, iced drinks, and long-term lifestyle aberrations, the body and mind lose their innate sense of order and intelligence, and the channels are thrown into chaos.

This little book is a plea for ecological and physiological sanity in an era of chaos. As David Krakauer of the Santa Fe Institute said, "intelligence means making hard problems easy."[2] Ministerial

---

2   See Paulson, S. (2015) *What is Genius? A Conversation with David Krakauer.* Nautilus. http://archive.ttbook.org/book/what-genius-conversation-david-krakauer.

fire is both complex and the essence of simplicity in medical and longevity practices. May it serve you well in recovering your own health and sanity, and may the warm embers of your own ministerial fire bring long life and spread to your family, community, bioregion, and the entire world.

Afterword

Reflecting on the Long/Short Journey

After more than two years of writing, this small book is now finally near the finish line. As with my first book it is a boiled-down, condensed work, inspired by the examples given me by David Weininger (representing a large amount of information as a small amount of information) and Albert Einstein ("make things as simple as possible, but no simpler"). It turns out that was a much more difficult task than I expected with a topic such as ministerial fire. Writing during a pandemic meant no physical contact or live meetings with my editors or colleagues, and a number of demands on my personal life that made writing more sporadic than usual. Also, unlike direct commentaries on texts such as the *Nán Jīng* 難經 (which I will continue with my next book), this required a broad range of reading and research. Ministerial fire, as an essential principle and force in Chinese medicine and philosophy, has been approached from multiple and sometimes contradictory angles throughout its history. Like fire itself, this principle is very fluid, ever changing, and hard to lock down. This book, in its finished form, is hardly a historical survey (there are many sources for this), or a clinical manual. Rather, it is a reflection, through my own eyes as an ongoing teacher and student of the medicine, on how I view the world and the clinical setting. I hope that I have succeeded in this task. Please utilize this book as a meditation on the profound ecological, medical, and philosophical nature of Chinese medicine and allow it to be absorbed into your consciousness, then reflect outwards to yourself, family, community, and patients. We need the ecological message of Chinese medicine more than ever.

APPENDIX I

Musings on the Pandemic
Epidemics and Ministerial Fire

The air has changed… It began as a trip to Yosemite National Park in September 2019. It was a sublime trip into the heart of these noble mountains and parkland, but it felt like a goodbye. Our last stop was at the Mariposa Sequoia Grove, a stately, ancient grove of trees.[1] Recently, this grove had been upgraded with new walkways, safeguards, and guided tours, but was still endangered in the foreseeable future by climate change. As my wife Edith and I left the park, I witnessed countless miles of dead forests and beetle-damaged trees, burnt out by raging fires just a few years ago. As we approached the Central Valley, a thick layer of smog and dust was lurking overhead in the sticky heat.[2]

Not long after our visit, severe fires devastated Northern California for the second year in a row, leading to serious air pollution in the San Francisco Bay area. Then, the Amazon suffered catastrophic fires. Soon afterwards, vast fires consumed

---

1   See Lahr, K. (2020) *Watching the Giant Sequoias Die*. Slate, April 21. https://slate.com/technology/2020/04/climate-change-giant-sequoias.html.
2   Meadows, M. (2021) *What I Saw in Yosemite Was Devastating*. New York Times, July 22. www.nytimes.com/2021/07/22/opinion/yosemite-west-coast-smoke.html?action=click&module=Opinion&pgtype=Homepage.

the bush country of Australia, killing approximately 1.25 billion native animals in the process. All the while, Australia's government downplayed the threat of climate change, despite record heat waves and drought. As the government is largely funded by the fossil fuel industry, recent coal mines had been approved, allowing fossil fuels to be shipped to China and other locales from a port dangerously close to the Great Coral Reef.[3] Two summers later, in late July 2021, we saw record heat in the Pacific Northwest, a massive, million-acre fire in Oregon that shrouded the East Coast in smoke and haze, three-million-acre fires in Siberia, extreme dryness with water shortages in California and Iran, and floods in Germany and Henan Province in China. The COVID-19 pandemic continues sporadically, with new variants, and plastic pollution becomes more pervasive. Our yin fire petroleum civilization seems to have turned a corner, where heaven and earth are unable to neutralize the toxic pollution generated by this civilization that relies on coal tar chemistry for its fuel, energy, heating, cooking, drugs, packaging, building materials, and insulation. A major turning point has been reached. While more and more people are recognizing and seeing the effects of climate change, the connection with pandemics has not yet been made. If the qi of heaven and earth are obscured, it leaves a *xū* 虛/vacuum that can easily be filled by *xié qì* 邪氣/evil qi.

I taught a seminar in San Jose in mid-December 2019, then spent time in Berkeley and San Francisco, where I got deeply chilled by unusually cold weather while staying in a small cottage that was poorly heated. On my return to San Diego, I took a walk on the beach at Torrey Pines, where the weather was usually cold, windy and damp, like much of this past winter. From my journal (December 2019):

---

3   The recent COVID-19 pandemic has led to some regeneration of the Great Barrier Reef and other coral reefs due to the reduction of human industrial activities.

Here in Southern California, the houses are not well heated, and the walls are thin, so the cold and damp permeate. This winter has been cold damp and windy, the ground wet from recent heavy rains. A chill arose from the ocean as I walked, and everyone I met seemed to be suffering from *shānghán* 傷寒/*zhòng fēng* 中風. Cold dribbling snivel, scratchy throat, loose, heated bowel movements, and today aches, kidney yang agitated and counter flowing with back pain. The mountains are covered with snow, and more storms are forecast.

Several weeks later, Edith and I took a trip to Hawaii for her birthday. By then, news of a strange epidemic in the Wuhan region of China had appeared. I noticed that even in Hawaii, the air seemed strange, as if permeated by an invisible imbalance, an evil qi spreading through the atmosphere. It felt to me as if a threshold in a natural balance had been reached, and that yin and yang, five phases and seasonal qi were in contention with each other. We noted that there was a feeling of unreality being in Hawaii, as if we were experiencing something that had changed, that looked and felt the same, but was utterly different—so much so, that we cut our vacation short and hurried back home. In a recent conversation with Heiner Fruehauf, Founding Professor of Chinese philosophy and herbs at the National College of Naturopathic Medicine in Portland, Oregon, he noted that this is exactly what ancient physicians must have meant in describing their experience of *yì qì* 疫氣/pestilential qi.[4]

Soon after, in March, I took one more trip to Berkeley to teach. This happened to be at the same time that a cruise ship

---

4 Recent research connects the lack of sunspot activity with an increase of pathogens in the stratosphere, which can descend to the immediate atmosphere that can affect humanity, especially in areas with high air pollution, or in dust clouds that blow from the Arabian subcontinent across the Atlantic Ocean, or descend to high altitude regions such as the Himalayas that then come down the mountains and cross China.

had docked in Oakland with several passengers infected with this strange new pathogen, on full moon, Purim time. Intuitively, I felt as if I needed to cancel a seminar the following weekend in San Jose, so I taught remotely for the first time. During the last hours of my seminar, the school was locked down and the remaining teachers and students were forced to leave. The following week, I made the decision to close my practice, two weeks before Passover began. Then daily life made its unspeakable shift into isolation, and everything shut down.

It is strange now, as I write this chapter (in March 2020, when people were staying at home and isolating), how the air is much clearer, but permeated with a yang pathogen that has spread throughout the world. This pathogen is spreading at rapid speed, as if *juéyīn* 厥陰's restraining gate was broken, and a downpour, a flood, was released. The birds sing, the flowers bloom, but on a visit to our local mountains, our trees are also dying or damaged.[5]

While preparing to return to clinical practice, I immersed myself in the medical classics, including the pulse chapters of Chéng Wújǐ's 成無己's *Shānghán Lùn* 傷寒論, the *Língshū*, *wǔ yùn liù qì* 五運六氣/five movements, and the six qi chapters of *Sùwèn* 素問. This was in between hiking, qi gong, yoga, eating lots of fermented foods such as miso and pickled vegetables, high fiber foods such as whole grains and leafy green vegetables, medicinal mushrooms such as *líng zhī* 靈芝/ganoderma, *dōng chóng xià cǎo* 冬蟲夏草/cordyceps, Chinese herbal formulas as needed, and treating myself with acupuncture and moxibustion. That is, of course, when not trying to transform panic and worry into tranquility, which consumes a great deal of qi. The inner transformation really is about mastering fire and water, *shàoyīn* 少陰, ministerial and sovereign fire.

---

5   Six months later, California has been beset by fires again in August and September. Today, smoke obscures the skies in San Diego, and parts of the city have had the highest temperatures ever recorded.

Perhaps it was just this period of learning I needed to be able to prepare such a book about ministerial fire, and really have it be my own work rather than the reportage of others' experiences. You can imagine how exciting this is for me. A colleague in Hong Kong sent me these articles. Now I've been able to put all the pieces together—how I sensed the toxic qi in the air in Hawaii, the descriptions in Navajo and Tibetan culture of pathogenic life forms in the air, and what Chinese medicine calls pestilential qi that Wú Yòukě 吳又可 described in the Qing dynasty as "living between heaven and earth." The article "Sunspot cycle minima and pandemics: The case for vigilance?"[6] gives a scientific analysis of the effects of climate, weather, altitude and a lack of solar flares to cleanse the atmosphere. It suggests that during the solar minimum,[7] new biological entities, viruses, bacteria, and so on can emerge. These can enter the interplanetary magnetic field barrier and reach the stratosphere and are mostly controlled by meteorological events as they pass through the lowest region of the atmosphere. As these particles descend they are deposited where in the stratosphere is thinnest, which includes areas of China east of the Himalayan mountain range, thus making it common to see new or renewed viral diseases being recorded in those regions. It is also important to know that not every solar minimum will be associated with new epidemics or pathogens.

In Tibetan medicine, these virulent infectious diseases are called *nyen-rim* གཉན་རིམས. A few of these illnesses have the capacity to eliminate 25 percent of living beings on our planet, and infect the majority of human beings. Tibetan medicine states that there

---

6   Wickramasinghe, N.C., Steele, E.J., Wainwright, M., Tokoro, G., Fernando, M. & Qu, J. (2017) "Sunspot Cycle Minima and Pandemics: The Case for Vigilance?" *Journal of Astrobiology & Outreach*, 5(2), 1.

7   Period of low solar activity in the 11-year solar cycle of the Sun. During this time, sunspot and solar flare activity diminishes, and often does not occur for days at a time.

are two critical factors: 1) lack of moral behavior and ethics 2) diet and lifestyle not in accordance with time and season.[8] When *wèi qì* 衛氣, and *dà qì* 大氣, the great qi of the air and sky, are damaged, *yì qì* 疫氣/pestilential qi thrives between heaven and earth. If *shí qì* 时氣/seasonal qi is out of order, the seasons arrive too early, too late, are too hot or too cold, too wet or too dry, and based on local climate norms, *wēn yì* 瘟疫/warm epidemics thrive. Unpredictable disease progressions occur in epidemics.

Viruses are expressions of intelligences in nature, even though they are simple packets of DNA/RNA that somehow know how to attach to hosts and replicate. They only become "living" when attaching themselves to the qi/life force of sentient life forms, whether plant, animal, or human. They have co-evolved with human beings, making it difficult to make vaccines and pharmaceutical treatments (as with SARS, HIV, and other viral disorders). Natural disasters, fires, wars, and famines create the conditions where these disease factors can proliferate. Another factor is that decreased sunspot activity fails to cleanse the atmosphere from microorganisms. As the great Japanese natural physician Masahilo Nakazono said, "we cannot kill anything in creation, we can try to destroy it, but it will just come back in another form."[9] If we do not consider the wider picture, specifically ecological, socioeconomic, and climactic factors, we will only see new pandemics and exotic pathogens develop.

---

8   See Andersson, E.J. (2020) *Tibetan Medicine and Covid-19*. Shrīmālā, November 6. www.shrimala.com/blog/tibetan-medicine-and-covid-19.

9   Nakazono, M. (1985) *A Guide to Inochi Medicine*. Kototama Institute.

Dìng Zhì Wán 定志丸 and Ministerial Fire

Ministerial fire has some unique expressions in the Chinese medical literature, one of them having to do with issues of heart and gall bladder vacuity. In *Sùwèn* 素問 8, the heart has the charge of the official functioning as "the ruler." If the ruler is enlightened, his subjects will be at peace. If the ruler is not enlightened, then all 12 officials will be in danger. In the same chapter, it states that the gall bladder is the official functioning as the "rectifier, and that decisions and judgments originate in it." According to *Nàn Jīng* 難經 42, the gall bladder stores and drains bile, and "is filled with three *gè* 個 of essence." Since the gall bladder is *shàoyáng* 少陽, and circulates ministerial fire, it has a direct influence on the heart/ruler, and stabilizes the sovereign fire.

In *Sùwèn* 47, "gall bladder solitary heat disease" (*dǎn dān* 膽癉), is discussed with a primary symptom of bitter taste. It is treated with GB 34 (*yáng líng quán* 陽陵泉). As rectifier, and decision-maker, the gall bladder advises the liver in making decisions. When the patient has "frequently planned and deliberated without reaching a decision," this is a sign that the gall bladder qi (膽虛氣) is vacuous. According to Zhāng Zhìcōng 張志聰, this means that liver qi is blocked and gall bladder qi depleted. This, in turn, can lead to the ministerial fire flaring upwards, producing evil heat.

In the past 16 months, since the beginning of the COVID-19 epidemic, I have seen an unusual percentage of patients with elevated, wiry left *cùn* 寸/inch and *guān* 關/gate pulses, indicating heart/gall bladder disharmonies. These often present with flaring ministerial fire disturbing the upper burner and the *shén* 神/spirit. Among the most important formula strategies, *dìng zhì wán* 定志丸/settle the will pill can be utilized to stabilize and calm the *hún* 魂/ethereal soul and *shén* to excellent effect. Contemplation of the mechanics of this formula and its modification reveals much about the relevance of ministerial fire in pathologies that include a *shén* component.

In the *Qiān Jīn Yào Fāng* 千金要方/*Prescriptions Worth 1000 Pieces of Gold* Sūn Sīmiǎo 孫思邈 writes the following about *dìng zhì wán*/settle the will pill: "It treats heart qi insufficiency and insufficiency of the five yin viscera. If severe, there will be damage from anxiety and sorrow and sudden forgetfulness." This formula supplements the heart (*xīn* 心) and boosts wisdom (*zhì* 志), settles timidity, and quiets the spirit. It governs the treatment of heart timidity with tendency to fear. The patient is not peaceful at night and unable to sleep, with disquietude when lying down. When the heart qi is insufficient, the heart spirit is deprived of nourishment. Therefore, there is heart timidity and a tendency to fear. The treatment strategy must supplement the heart and boost intelligence, quiet the spirit, and settle the will.

The sovereign medicinal, *rén shēn* 人參/ginseng radix, calms the spirit, nourishes the heart, boosts intelligence, and checks fright palpitations. It is sweet and cool in nature, and slightly bitter. When in its prepared form as *hóng rén shēn* 红人參/red ginseng it is warmer in nature and used for yang vacuity. In the *Shén Nóng Běncǎo Jīng* 神農本草經/*Divine Farmer's Materia Medica*, *rén shēn* is said to "supplementing the five zang organs, calming the essence spirit(s) and settle the *hún* and *pò* souls, stopping fright palpitations, expelling evil qì, brighten the eyes, and open the heart and boosting wisdom.[1]

When I prescribe *dìng zhì wán*, I will often substitute *fú líng* 茯苓/poria with *fú shēn* 茯神/poria sclerotium pararadicis, the portion connected to the pine root which is said to have a stronger spirit-calming effect. Its nature is sweet/bland, and neutral and in the *Qiān Jīn Yào Fāng*, Sūn Sīmiǎo writes, *fú shēn* treats:

> counterflow qi in the chest and rib-sides, anxiety and hatred, fright evils and fear palpitations, binding pain below the heart, [aversion to] cold and heat [effusion], vexation and fullness, cough with counterflow, parched mouth and dry tongue. Disinhibits urine. When taken over a long period, it quiets the ethereal soul, nourishes the spirit, and extends the years.[2]

Yuǎn zhì 遠志/polygalae radix calms the *shén*/spirit, and has the function of " treats counterflow cough and damage to the center; supplements insufficiency; gets rid of evil qì; disinhibits the Nine Orifices; boosts wisdom; makes the ears and eyes sharp and bright; staves off forgetfulness; strengthens the will; and multiplies strength."[3] *Shí chāng pú* 石菖蒲/acori tatarinowii rhizoma, treats "wind-cold and damp-related impediment, and counterflow cough with ascent of qì; opens up the apertures of the heart; supplements the five zàng organs; unclogs the Nine Orifices; brightens the ears and eyes; and makes the sound of the voice come forth. Consumed over a long time, it lightens the body, states off forgetfulness and confusion, and extends the years."[4] When these four medicinals

1   Wilms, S (2017) *The Divine Farmer's Classic of Materia Medica Shen Nong Bencao Jing*. Portland, OR: Happy Goat Productions, pp. 23.

2   Wilms, S (2008) *Bèi Jí Qiān Jīn Yào Fāng Essential Prescriptions Worth a Thousand Pieces of Gold for Every Emergency Volumes 2-4*. Corbett, OR: Happy Goat Productions, pp. 570.

3   Wilms, S (2017) *The Divine Farmer's Classic of Materia Medica Shen Nong Bencao Jing*. Portland, OR: Happy Goat Productions, pp. 61.

4   Ibid. pp. 35.

are used together, they have an excellent effect on the mind and body. Similar to *suān zǎo rén tāng* 酸棗仁湯/Zizyphus Jujube Decoction, *dìng zhì wán* calms the spirit and benefits sleep, but it also strengthens the heart as well.

The gall bladder, associated with the foot *shàoyáng* 少陽 channel, has wide-reaching effects on the body, emotions, and personality. According to *Sùwèn*, it is responsible for the decision-making capacity, and, in fact, *dǎn* 膽 also translates as audacity or courage in classical Chinese philosophical texts. The *shàoyáng* governs the movement and circulation of ministerial fire, and when the ministerial fire loses the regulation of the *shàoyáng*/gall bladder, emotions, heat and cold, and symptoms in general become changeable and erratic. The ministerial fire is erratic, leading to a poor distribution of heat and cold. When the ministerial fire is depleted, we must use the treatment method of *wēn dǎn* 溫膽/ warming the gall bladder.

Dìng zhì wán anchors the heart *shén*, dispels phlegm, opens the heart portals, and warms and anchors gall bladder qi and ministerial fire. Therefore, we use this formula, along with such formulas as *wēn dǎn tang* 溫膽湯/gall bladder warming decoction and *shí wèi wēn dǎn tang* 十味溫膽湯/ten-ingredient gall bladder-warming decoction to secure the ministerial fire and restore stability to the *hún* and *shén*. If *dìng zhì wán* is combined with *wēn dǎn tang* or *shí wèi wēn dǎn tang*, it is even more supportive of *shàoyáng*/ gall bladder ministerial fire. It helps with the decision-making capabilities of the "general/rectifier," as we saw in *Sùwèn* 8

According to Stephen Cowan, *dìng* 定/stabilization can be seen as "a kind of footing, foundation, equilibrium, or weathervane." Daniel Schrier adds that *dìng* 定 is a homophone with *dǐng* 鼎/ cauldron, a three-footed bronze vessel/cauldron used for cooking and/or making ritual offerings to the gods and ancestors. *Dǐng* 鼎 is represented in the *Yìjīng* 易經 as hexagram 50. The symbol is constructed of fire ☲ above wind ☴. The symbol is about the transformation of things, by depicting wind/wood as it feeds the fire to bring about growth, inspiration, and transformation towards personal and spiritual evolution. In *nèi dān* 內丹 practices, the *dǐng* 鼎 is situated in center of the lower *dān tián* 丹田. The three legs can symbolizes the three treasures of *jīng* 精, *qì* 氣, and *shén* 神. Like a cauldron, these three energetic substances are combined and transformed or "cooked" to initiate change and to elevate us from the mundane to spiritual.

It is interesting when one examines the character of the heart (*xīn* 心), we see three strokes at the bottom which could resemble the three legs of the *dǐng*. The heart is often described as an "empty vessel" so as to be capable of receiving what it is being poured in so that one can connect with the divine brilliance around us.

In conclusion, *dìng zhì wán* is an important formula that works with the gall bladder/heart connections (*shàoyáng/shàoyīn*), ministerial and heart fire, and anchors the will while calming the *shén*/spirit. In studying this formula, we can gain new perspectives on the management and treatment of issues involving ministerial fire.

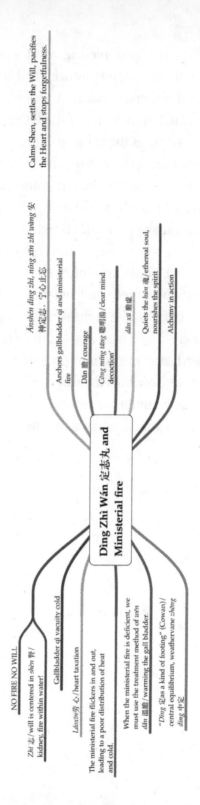

NO FIRE NO WILL

Zhi 志 / will is centered in *shèn* 腎 / kidney; fire within water!

Gallbladder qi vacuity cold

Láoxīnzǔ 心 / heart taxation

The ministerial fire flickers in and out, leading to a poor distribution of heat and cold.

When the ministerial fire is deficient, we must use the treatment method of *wēn dàn* 溫膽 / warming the gall bladder.

"*Dìng* 定as a kind of footing" (Cowan) / central equilibrium, weathervane *zhōng dìng* 中定

Dìng Zhì Wán 定志丸 and Ministerial fire

Ānshén dìng zhì, níng xīn zhì wàng 安神定志, 宁心止忘

Anchors gallbladder qi and ministerial fire

Dǎn 膽 / courage

Cōng míng tāng 聰明湯 / clear mind decoction'

dǎn xū 膽虛

Quiets the *hún* 魂 / ethereal soul, nourishes the spirit

Alchemy in action

Calms Shen, settles the Will, pacifies the Heart and stops forgetfulness.

Dìng Zhì Wán and Ministerial Fire

Blueprints and Charts From Z'ev's Notebook

Mindmaps for Pattern-Based Thinking

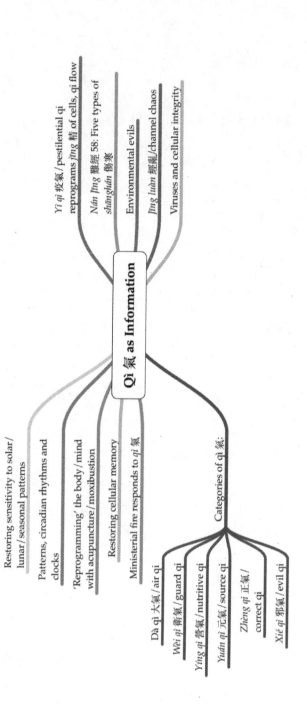

Qi as Information

Fire, Qi, Location, Time
Shao Yin and Ministerial Fire

Central node: **Fire, Qi, Location, Time**

Right branches:
- *Jìn* 晉 - hexagram 35 晉
- *Xīn* 心 / Heart / mind
- Reversal and yang qi
- *Shàoyīn* 少陰 pivot
- *Shàoyáng* 少陽 / Gall Bladder
- *Shàoyáng* 少陽 pivot
- Fire and water
- Daytime *tàiyáng* 太陽 - Sun rising over the earth

Left branches:
- Night / yin - Sun sinking under the earth
- *Míng yí* 明夷 - hexagram 36 夷
- *Tàiyáng* 太陽 / *shàoyīn* 少陰 relationship
- *Jīng* 精 / *shén* 神 / 身体 *shàoyīn* 少陰
- Ministerial fire / *shén* tǐ 身体 / physiology
- Sovereign fire / illumination
- *Tàiyáng* 太陽 morning / *shàoyīn* 少陰 nighttime

Autoimmunity & the Chinese Ecological Model

- internal taxation/external hyperactivity
- Mind pushing body with hyper work schedule
- External yang battle exhausting internal resources
- Essence no longer anchors yin and yang separation
- Yin depleting hyperactivity at yang aspect shàoyīn

- mǎ huáng zhī mǔ sháo yào tāng 麻黄鳞知母芍藥湯
- Jué 絕: "not completely filling out one's own space" (Hood)
- Yang within yin...use warm acrid herbs inside yin protective herbs fù zǐ 附子/aconiti radix lateralis/bái sháo 白芍/paeoniae radix alba
- Bioengineering model vs. Chinese medicine ecological model
- Autoimmune disease mirrors climate change issues
- Forest fires generate their own weather: thunderstorms and wind

Autoimmunity/Chinese Ecological Model

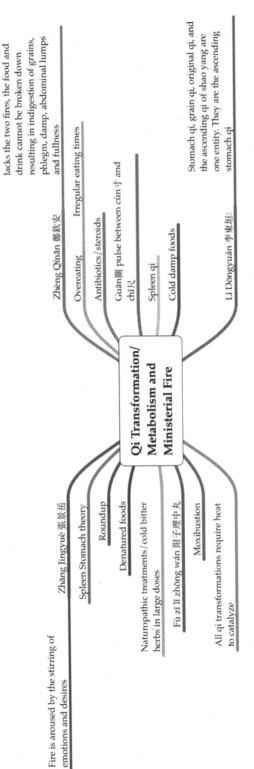

Qi Transformation/Metabolism and Ministerial Fire

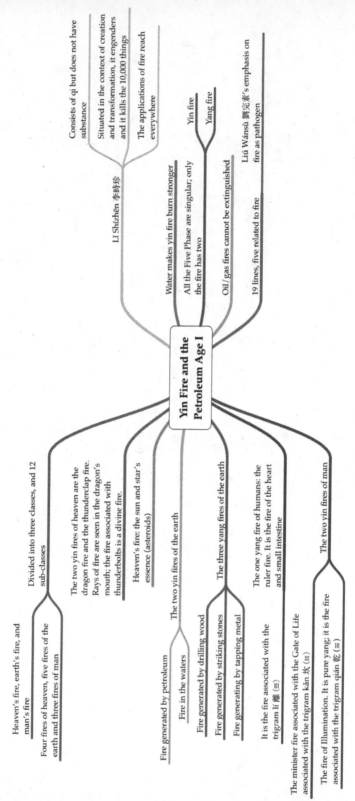

Yin Fire and the Petroleum Age

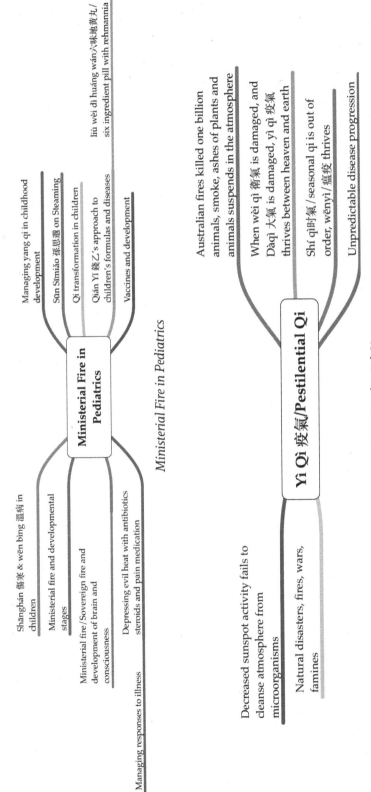

Ministerial Fire in Pediatrics

Ministerial Fire in Pediatrics

- Managing yang qi in childhood development
- Sūn Sīmiǎo 孫思邈 on Steaming
- Qi transformation in children
- Qián Yǐ 錢乙's approach to children's formulas and diseases
- Vaccines and development

- Shānghán 傷寒 & wēn bìng 溫病 in children
- Ministerial fire and developmental stages
- Ministerial fire/Sovereign fire and development of brain and consciousness
- Depressing evil heat with antibiotics steroids and pain medication
- Managing responses to illness

Ministerial Fire in Pediatrics

Yi Qi Pestilential Qi

Yì Qì 疫氣/Pestilential Qi

- Australian fires killed one billion animals, smoke, ashes of plants and animals suspends in the atmosphere
- When wèi qì 衛氣 is damaged, and Dàqì 大氣 is damaged, yì qì 疫氣 thrives between heaven and earth
- Shí qì时气/ seasonal qi is out of order, wēnyì / 瘟疫 thrives
- Unpredictable disease progression

- Decreased sunspot activity fails to cleanse atmosphere from microorganisms
- Natural disasters, fires, wars, famines

Yì Qì 疫氣 Pestilential Qi

Index